Experimental and Clinical Treatment of Subarachnoid Hemorrhage after Rupture of Saccular Intracranial Aneurysms

Experimental and Clinical Treatment of Subarachnoid Hemorrhage after Rupture of Saccular Intracranial Aneurysms

Editors

Serge Marbacher
John H. Zhang

MDPI • Basel • Beijing • Wuhan • Barcelona • Belgrade • Manchester • Tokyo • Cluj • Tianjin

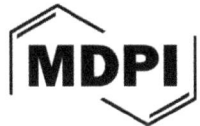

Editors
Serge Marbacher
Kantonsspital Aarau
Switzerland

John H. Zhang
Loma Linda University
USA

Editorial Office
MDPI
St. Alban-Anlage 66
4052 Basel, Switzerland

This is a reprint of articles from the Special Issue published online in the open access journal *Brain Sciences* (ISSN 2076-3425) (available at: https://www.mdpi.com/journal/brainsci/special_issues/Subarachnoid_Hemorrhage).

For citation purposes, cite each article independently as indicated on the article page online and as indicated below:

LastName, A.A.; LastName, B.B.; LastName, C.C. Article Title. *Journal Name* **Year**, *Article Number*, Page Range.

ISBN 978-3-03943-154-0 (Hbk)
ISBN 978-3-03943-155-7 (PDF)

Cover image courtesy of Serge Marbacher.

© 2020 by the authors. Articles in this book are Open Access and distributed under the Creative Commons Attribution (CC BY) license, which allows users to download, copy and build upon published articles, as long as the author and publisher are properly credited, which ensures maximum dissemination and a wider impact of our publications.

The book as a whole is distributed by MDPI under the terms and conditions of the Creative Commons license CC BY-NC-ND.

Contents

About the Editors . . . . **vii**

Serge Marbacher and John H. Zhang
Experimental and Clinical Treatment of Subarachnoid Hemorrhage after the Rupture of Saccular Intracranial Aneurysms
Reprinted from: *Brain Sci.* **2020**, *10*, 371, doi:10.3390/brainsci10060371 . . . . **1**

Mieko Oka, Isao Ono, Kampei Shimizu, Mika Kushamae, Haruka Miyata, Takakazu Kawamata and Tomohiro Aoki
The Bilateral Ovariectomy in a Female Animal Exacerbates the Pathogenesis of an Intracranial Aneurysm
Reprinted from: *Brain Sci.* **2020**, *10*, 335, doi:10.3390/brainsci10060335 . . . . **3**

Jenny C. Kienzler, Michael Diepers, Serge Marbacher, Luca Remonda and Javier Fandino
Endovascular Temporary Balloon Occlusion for Microsurgical Clipping of Posterior Circulation Aneurysms
Reprinted from: *Brain Sci.* **2020**, *10*, 334, doi:10.3390/brainsci10060334 . . . . **15**

Basil Erwin Grüter, Stefan Wanderer, Fabio Strange, Sivani Sivanrupan, Michael von Gunten, Hans Rudolf Widmer, Daniel Coluccia, Lukas Andereggen, Javier Fandino and Serge Marbacher
Comparison of Aneurysm Patency and Mural Inflammation in an Arterial Rabbit Sidewall and Bifurcation Aneurysm Model under Consideration of Different Wall Conditions
Reprinted from: *Brain Sci.* **2020**, *10*, 197, doi:10.3390/brainsci10040197 . . . . **35**

Davide Marco Croci, Stefan Wanderer, Fabio Strange, Basil E. Grüter, Daniela Casoni, Sivani Sivanrupan, Hans Rudolf Widmer, Stefano Di Santo, Javier Fandino, Luigi Mariani and Serge Marbacher
Systemic and CSF Interleukin-1α Expression in a Rabbit Closed Cranium Subarachnoid Hemorrhage Model: An Exploratory Study
Reprinted from: *Brain Sci.* **2019**, *9*, 249, doi:10.3390/brainsci9100249 . . . . **47**

Stefan Wanderer, Basil E. Grüter, Fabio Strange, Sivani Sivanrupan, Stefano Di Santo, Hans Rudolf Widmer, Javier Fandino, Serge Marbacher and Lukas Andereggen
The Role of Sartans in the Treatment of Stroke and Subarachnoid Hemorrhage: A Narrative Review of Preclinical and Clinical Studies
Reprinted from: *Brain Sci.* **2020**, *10*, 153, doi:10.3390/brainsci10030153 . . . . **57**

Fabio Strange, Basil E Grüter, Javier Fandino and Serge Marbacher
Preclinical Intracranial Aneurysm Models: A Systematic Review
Reprinted from: *Brain Sci.* **2020**, *10*, 134, doi:10.3390/brainsci10030134 . . . . **83**

Serge Marbacher, Stefan Wanderer, Fabio Strange, Basil E. Grüter and Javier Fandino
Saccular Aneurysm Models Featuring Growth and Rupture: A Systematic Review
Reprinted from: *Brain Sci.* **2020**, *10*, 101, doi:10.3390/brainsci10020101 . . . . **99**

Chan-Hyuk Park, Hyeong Ryu, Chang-Hwan Kim, Kyung-Lim Joa, Myeong-Ok Kim and Han-Young Jung
Injury of Corticospinal Tract in a Patient with Subarachnoid Hemorrhage as Determined by Diffusion Tensor Tractography: A Case Report
Reprinted from: *Brain Sci.* **2020**, *10*, 177, doi:10.3390/brainsci10030177 . . . . **109**

Meng-Yu Wu, Ching-Hsiang Lin, Yueh-Tseng Hou, Po-Chen Lin, Giou-Teng Yiang, Yueh-Cheng Tien and Hsiao-Ching Yeh
Syncope as Initial Presentation in an Undifferentiated Type Acute Myeloid Leukemia Patient with Acute Intracranial Hemorrhage
Reprinted from: *Brain Sci.* **2019**, *9*, 207, doi:10.3390/brainsci9080207 . . . . **117**

About the Editors

Serge Marbacher (PD, MD, PhD) https://www.ksa.ch/sites/default/files/cms/neurochirurgie/docs/cv-marbac

John H. Zhang The clinically related basic science research in the Zhang Neuroscience Research Laboratories focuses on cerebral vascular diseases (stroke). The main research direction in the Zhang Laboratory is focused on the ischemic and hemorrhagic stroke, as well as global cerebral ischemia, neonatal hypoxia, and neurological complications of neurosurgery and anesthesia. Animal models of the above mentioned neurological disorders are currently employed in the studies of cerebral physiology including the blood–brain barrier, brain edema, cerebral blood flow and intracranial pressure, cerebral morphology, especially immunohistochemistry, molecular biology, neuro-imaging, neurological and neurobehavioral functional testing. The main focus of research interests is cerebral vascular biology, neuroprotective strategies, gene therapy, signaling pathways, apoptosis, and hyperbaric medicine.

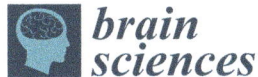

Editorial

Experimental and Clinical Treatment of Subarachnoid Hemorrhage after the Rupture of Saccular Intracranial Aneurysms

Serge Marbacher [1,2,*] and John H. Zhang [3]

1. Department of Neurosurgery, Kantonsspital Aarau, 5000 Aarau, Switzerland
2. Cerebrovascular Research Group, Neurosurgery, Department for BioMedical Research, University of Bern, 3010 Bern, Switzerland
3. Departments of Neurosurgery, Physiology, and Anesthesiology, Loma Linda University School of Medicine, Loma Linda, CA 92354, USA; jhzhang@llu.edu
* Correspondence: serge.marbacher@ksa.ch or neurosurgery@ksa.ch

Received: 9 June 2020; Accepted: 10 June 2020; Published: 15 June 2020

The Special Issue "Experimental and Clinical Treatment of Subarachnoid Hemorrhage after the Rupture of Saccular Intracranial Aneurysms" provides an excellent insight into the many facets of aneurysmal subarachnoid hemorrhage. The call for papers on this topic was met with a great response by researchers and clinicians from all over the world. Among 16 basic science and clinical research submissions, our editorial team selected nine articles for publication after extensive peer review, which included three original papers [1–3], three reviews [4–6], two case reports [7,8] and one technical note [9]. The remaining seven papers were not included, thus yielding a 44% rejection rate.

Two of the three review articles systematically summarize the current literature on preclinical intracranial and extracranial aneurysm models [4,5]. In a review article on preclinical intracranial aneurysm models, Strange et al. provides a comprehensive summary of the multitude of available models to study various aspects of aneurysm formation, growth, and rupture; it serves as an extremely useful compendium for researchers entering this field of research [5]. The review article on preclinical extracranial aneurysm models focuses on a small subgroup of models that feature growth and eventually rupture [4,10]. These models hold special interest for researchers testing novel endovascular devices as the last step before initiating a first clinical trial.

In an original study using an extracranial aneurysm model in rabbits, researchers confirmed that, under flow conditions in a bifurcation aneurysm, the organization of an intraluminal thrombus was strongly dependent on the condition of the aneurysm wall [2]. In another original work featuring an intracranial aneurysm model on rats, authors investigated how sex hormones influence the inflammatory reactions in the aneurysm walls and affect the endothelial cells of the vascular walls [3]. The three original papers are basic research; the case studies and technical note are clinical papers [7–9].

This Special Issue represents a compilation of important clinical and preclinical papers by innovative researchers that enhance our understanding about subarachnoid hemorrhage and intracranial aneurysms. Their research inspires commitment in our future research for our patients who face these devastating conditions.

Acknowledgments: We express our gratitude and recognition to all reviewers who participated in the review process. Their commitment to critically evaluate and comment on the manuscripts substantially improved each article and enhanced the overall quality of this special issue. We thank Mary Kemper for editing.

Conflicts of Interest: The authors declare that they have no conflict of interest.

References

1. Croci, D.M.; Wanderer, S.; Strange, F.; Grüter, B.E.; Casoni, D.; Sivanrupan, S.; Widmer, H.R.; Di Santo, S.; Fandino, J.; Mariani, L.; et al. Systemic and CSF Interleukin-1alpha Expression in a Rabbit Closed Cranium Subarachnoid Hemorrhage Model: An Exploratory Study. *Brain Sci.* **2019**, *9*, 249. [CrossRef] [PubMed]
2. Grüter, B.E.; Wanderer, S.; Strange, F.; Sivanrupan, S.; von Gunten, M.; Widmer, H.R.; Coluccia, D.; Andereggen, L.; Fandino, J.; Marbacher, S. Comparison of Aneurysm Patency and Mural Inflammation in an Arterial Rabbit Sidewall and Bifurcation Aneurysm Model under Consideration of Different Wall Conditions. *Brain Sci.* **2020**, *10*, 197. [CrossRef] [PubMed]
3. Oka, M.; Ono, I.; Shimizu, K.; Kushamae, M.; Miyata, H.; Kawamata, T.; Aoki, T. The Bilateral Ovariectomy in a Female Animal Exacerbates the Pathogenesis of an Intracranial Aneurysm. *Brain Sci.* **2020**, *10*, 335. [CrossRef] [PubMed]
4. Marbacher, S.; Strange, F.; Frosen, J.; Fandino, J. Preclinical extracranial aneurysm models for the study and treatment of brain aneurysms: A systematic review. *J. Cereb. Blood Flow Metab.* **2020**, *40*, 922–938. [CrossRef] [PubMed]
5. Strange, F.; Gruter, B.E.; Fandino, J.; Marbacher, S. Preclinical Intracranial Aneurysm Models: A Systematic Review. *Brain Sci.* **2020**, *10*, 134. [CrossRef] [PubMed]
6. Wanderer, S.; Grüter, B.E.; Strange, F.; Sivanrupan, S.; Di Santo, S.; Widmer, H.R.; Fandino, J.; Marbacher, S.; Andereggen, L. The Role of Sartans in the Treatment of Stroke and Subarachnoid Hemorrhage: A Narrative Review of Preclinical and Clinical Studies. *Brain Sci.* **2020**, *10*, 153. [CrossRef] [PubMed]
7. Park, C.H.; Ryu, H.; Kim, C.H.; Joa, K.L.; Kim, M.O.; Jung, H.Y. Injury of Corticospinal Tract in a Patient with Subarachnoid Hemorrhage as Determined by Diffusion Tensor Tractography: A Case Report. *Brain Sci.* **2020**, *10*, 177. [CrossRef] [PubMed]
8. Wu, M.Y.; Lin, C.H.; Hou, Y.T.; Lin, P.C.; Yiang, G.T.; Tien, Y.C.; Yeh, H.C. Syncope as Initial Presentation in an Undifferentiated Type Acute Myeloid Leukemia Patient with Acute Intracranial Hemorrhage. *Brain Sci.* **2019**, *9*, 207. [CrossRef] [PubMed]
9. Kienzler, J.C.; Diepers, M.; Marbacher, S.; Remonda, L.; Fandino, J. Endovascular Temporary Balloon Occlusion for Microsurgical Clipping of Posterior Circulation Aneurysms. *Brain Sci.* **2020**, *10*, 334. [CrossRef] [PubMed]
10. Marbacher, S.; Wanderer, S.; Strange, F.; Gruter, B.E.; Fandino, J. Saccular Aneurysm Models Featuring Growth and Rupture: A Systematic Review. *Brain Sci.* **2020**, *10*, 101. [CrossRef] [PubMed]

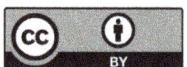

© 2020 by the authors. Licensee MDPI, Basel, Switzerland. This article is an open access article distributed under the terms and conditions of the Creative Commons Attribution (CC BY) license (http://creativecommons.org/licenses/by/4.0/).

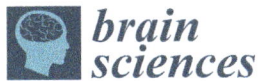

Article

The Bilateral Ovariectomy in a Female Animal Exacerbates the Pathogenesis of an Intracranial Aneurysm

Mieko Oka [1,2,3], Isao Ono [1,2,4], Kampei Shimizu [1,2,4], Mika Kushamae [1,2,5], Haruka Miyata [1,2,6], Takakazu Kawamata [3] and Tomohiro Aoki [1,2,*]

1. Department of Molecular Pharmacology, Research Institute, National Cerebral and Cardiovascular Center, Osaka 564-8565, Japan; happy.harmony.toto@gmail.com (M.O.); onoisao@kuhp.kyoto-u.ac.jp (I.O.); k.shimizu.830923@gmail.com (K.S.); marojiji9@yahoo.co.jp (M.K.); hmiyata27@gmail.com (H.M.)
2. Core Research for Evolutional Science and Technology (CREST) from Japan Agency for Medical Research and Development (AMED), National Cerebral and Cardiovascular Center, Osaka 564-8565, Japan
3. Department of Neurosurgery, Tokyo Women's Medical University, Tokyo 162-8666, Japan; tkawamata@twmu.ac.jp
4. Department of Neurosurgery, Kyoto University Graduate School of Medicine, Tokyo 606-8507, Japan
5. Department of Neurosurgery, Showa University, Tokyo 142-8666, Japan
6. Department of Neurosurgery, Shiga University of Medical Science, Shiga 520-2192, Japan
* Correspondence: tomoaoki@ncvc.go.jp; Tel.: +81-6-6170-1070 (ext. 31022)

Received: 24 April 2020; Accepted: 28 May 2020; Published: 31 May 2020

Abstract: Considering the poor outcome of subarachnoid hemorrhage (SAH) due to the rupture of intracranial aneurysms (IA), mechanisms underlying the pathogenesis of IAs, especially the rupture of lesions, should be clarified. In the present study, a rat model of IAs in which induced lesions spontaneously ruptured resulting in SAH was used. In this model, the combination of the female sex and the bilateral ovariectomy increased the incidence of SAH, similar to epidemiological evidence in human cases. Importantly, unruptured IA lesions induced in female animals with bilateral ovariectomy were histopathologically similar to ruptured ones in the presence of vasa vasorum and the accumulation of abundant inflammatory cells, suggesting the exacerbation of the disease. The post-stenotic dilatation of the carotid artery was disturbed by the bilateral ovariectomy in female rats, which was restored by hormone replacement therapy. The in vivo study thus suggested the protective effect of estrogen from the ovary on endothelial cells loaded by wall shear stress. β-estradiol or dihydrotestosterone also suppressed the lipopolysaccharide-induced expression of pro-inflammatory genes in cultured macrophages and neutrophils. The results of the present study have thus provided new insights about the process regulating the progression of the disease.

Keywords: intracranial aneurysm; subarachnoid hemorrhage; estrogen; female; endothelial cell; macrophage

---

1. Introduction

Considering the devastating outcome of subarachnoid hemorrhage (SAH) due to the rupture of an intracranial aneurysm (IA) [1,2], the development of a novel therapeutic strategy to prevent the rupture of IAs is mandatory for social health. Mechanisms underlying the rupture of lesions should, therefore, be clarified. Thus, we attempted to find a cue from well-established epidemiological evidence. Epidemiological studies have consistently demonstrated a higher incidence of SAH in older females or postmenopausal females [3–8]. Based on the necessity of clarifying underlying mechanisms of the rupture of IAs, we examined whether sex difference is indeed present, and if present, why, using the already-established animal model of IAs [9].

2. Materials and Methods

2.1. IA Models of Rats and Histological Analysis of Induced IA

All of the following experiments, including animal care and use, complied with the National Institute of Health's Guide for the Care and Use of Laboratory Animals and complied with the National Institute of Health's Guide for the Care and Use of Laboratory Animals and were approved by the Institutional Animal Care and Use Committee of the National Cerebral and Cardiovascular Center (Approved number; #18010 and #19036). The present manuscript also adheres to the ARRIVE (Animal Research: Reporting of In Vivo Experiments) guidelines for reporting animal experiments.

Ten-week-old male or female Sprague–Dawley (SD) rats were purchased from Japan SLC (Slc:SD, Shizuoka, Japan) ($n = 62$ in total). Animals were maintained on a 12-h light/dark cycle, and had free access to feed and water. To induce IAs, the rats were subjected to ligation of the left carotid artery, the right external carotid artery and the right pterygopalatine artery, and systemic hypertension by the combination of a high salt diet and the ligation of the left renal artery under general anesthesia by the intraperitoneal injection of pentobarbital sodium (50 mg/kg, Somnopentyl, Kyoritsuseiyaku Corporation, Tokyo, Japan) and the inhalation of Isoflurane (1.5%–2%, #IYESC-0001, Pfizer Inc., New York, NY). In some female rats, the bilateral ovariectomy was also applied [9]. Immediately after the above surgical manipulations, animals were fed chow containing 8% sodium chloride and 0.12% 3-aminopropionitrile (#A0408, Tokyo Chemical Industry, Tokyo, Japan), an irreversible inhibitor of lysyl oxidase catalyzing the cross-linking of collagen and elastin. Animals that died within one week after the above surgical manipulations were excluded from the analyses. At 16 weeks after the surgical manipulations, blood pressure was measured by a tail-cuff method without any anesthesia and was calculated as an average of three measurements. Animals were then deeply anesthetized by an intraperitoneal injection of pentobarbital sodium (200 mg/kg), and transcardially perfused with 4% paraformaldehyde solution. The circle of Willis was then stripped from the brain surface and an IA lesion induced at the anterior communicating artery or the posterior communicating artery was dissected as a ruptured or unruptured lesion, according to the macroscopic observation of whether the clot or hemosiderin deposition was present around IA lesions. Here, ruptured IAs were exclusively induced at these sites examined in the model [9]. All the dead animals after at least one week of surgical manipulations were autopsied to examine the onset of SAH due to rupture of induced IAs. Histopathological examination was done after Elastica van Gieson, which visualizes the internal elastic lamina using 5-um-thick frozen sections. The size of induced lesions was analyzed using the slices with the maximum area selected from serial sections using ImageJ software (https://imagej.nih.gov/ij/index.html).

2.2. Immunohistochemistry

At the indicated period after the aneurysm induction, 5-μm-thick frozen sections were prepared. After blocking with 3% donkey serum (#AB_2337258, Jackson ImmunoResearch, Baltimore, MD, USA), slices were incubated with primary antibodies, followed by incubation with secondary antibodies conjugated with a fluorescence dye (Jackson ImmunoResearch). Finally, fluorescent images were acquired using a confocal fluorescence microscope system (FV1000 or FV3000, Olympus, Tokyo, Japan).

The following primary antibodies were used: mouse monoclonal anti-CD68 antibody (#ab31630, Abcam, Cambridge, UK), rabbit polyclonal anti-myeloperoxidase (MPO) antibody (#ab9535, Abcam), rabbit polyclonal anti-tumor necrosis factor (TNF)-alpha antibody (#ab6671, Abcam), mouse monoclonal anti-smooth muscle α-actin (SMA) antibody (#M0851, Dako, Agilent, Santa Clara, CA, USA).

The following secondary antibodies were used; Alexa Fluor 488-conjugated donkey anti-mouse IgG H&L antibody (#A21202, Thermo Fisher Scientific, Waltham, MA, USA), Alexa Fluor 488-conjugated donkey anti-rabbit IgG H&L antibody (#A21206, Thermo Fisher Scientific), Alexa Fluor 594-conjugated donkey anti-mouse IgG H&L antibody (#A21203, Thermo Fisher Scientific).

2.3. Stenosis Model of the Carotid Artery of a Rat

Female rats underwent a bilateral ovariectomy and sham operation, and were then maintained for 7 days before subjecting to the model. The left common carotid artery of rats was then ligated using a 10-0 nylon thread with 25 gauge needle put on the side of the artery and stenosis was established by removing only the needle [10,11]. The post-stenotic dilatation of the carotid artery was observed for 30 min after ligation.

2.4. Hormone Replacement Therapy

Estradiol valerate (1 mg/kg, #224136400 Pelanin Depot, Mochida Pharmaceutical Co., Ltd., Tokyo, Japan) was intramuscularly injected every 7 days in a female rat that underwent the bilateral ovariectomy.

2.5. Cell Line and Culture

RAW264.7 cell line (#TIB-71), used as a macrophage, and HL-60 cell line (#CCL-240), used as a neutrophil, were purchased from ATCC (Manassas, VA, USA) and maintained in Dulbecco's Modified Eagle's Medium (DMEM) (#044-32955, FUJIFILM Wako Pure Chemical Corporation, Osaka, Japan) supplemented with 10% or 20% fetal bovine serum (#FB-1365/500, Biosera, Nuaille, France), respectively.

2.6. Quantitative Real Time (RT)-PCR Analysis in Cultured Cells

RAW264.7 cells or HL-60 cells were pre-treated with β-estradiol (E2, 50 µg/mL, #E0025, Tokyo Chemical Industry) or 5α-Dihydrotestosterone (DHT, 50 µg/mL, #A0462, Tokyo Chemical Industry) for 24 h or 3 h, respectively. Cells were then stimulated with vehicle (Veh), LPS (1 µg/mL, #L2654, Sigma Aldrich, St. Louis, MO, USA) or TNF-α (100 ng/mL, R&D SYSTEMS, Minneapolis, MN, USA) for additional 60 min.

Total RNA was purified from stimulated cells and reverse-transcribed using a RNeasy Mini Kit (#74106, QIAGEN, Hilden, Germany) and a High-capacity cDNA Reverse Transcription Kit (#4368813, Life Technologies Corporation, Carlsbad, CA, USA), according to the manufacturers' instructions. For quantification of gene expression, quantitative RT-PCR was performed on a LightCycler 480 (Roche, Indianapolis, IN, USA) with a TB Green Premix Ex Taq II (#RR820, TAKARA BIO INC., Shiga, Japan). Expression of *Actb* (a gene coding β-actin) in experiments using the RAW264.7 cell line, or *ACTB* in experiments using the HL-60 cell line, were used as internal controls. For quantitation, the second derivative maximum method was used for determining the crossing point.

Primer sets used are listed as follows: forward 5′-CACCTCAGGGAAGAATCTGG-3′ and reverse 5′-CATTCCTGAGTTCTGCAAAGG-3′ for *Tnf*; forward 5′-AAAGGGAGCTCCTTAACATGC-3′ and reverse 5′-CTTCCTGGGAAACAACAGTGG-3′ for *Il1b*; forward 5′-AATGATGTGTACGGCTTCAGG-3′ and reverse 5′-CTGTACAAGCAGTGGCAAAGG-3′ for *Ptgs2* (a gene encoding cyclooxygenase-2 (COX-2)); forward 5′-GCACAGACCTCTCTCTTGAGC-3′ and reverse 5′-ACCTGCTGCTGCTACTCATTCACC-3′ for *Ccl2* (a gene encoding monocyte chemoattractant protein-1 (MCP-1)); 5′-ACGACCAGAGGCATACAGGGA-3′ and 5′-CCCTAAGGCCAACCGTGAAA-3′ for *Actb*; forward 5′-TCAGCAATGAGTGACAGTTGG-3′ and reverse 5′-ATAGGCTGTTCCCATGTAGCC-3′ for *TNF*; forward 5′-CAAGCTGGAATTTGAGTCGC-3′ and reverse 5′-ATTCAGCACAGGACTCTCTGG-3′ for *IL1B*; forward 5′-ACACCCTCTATCACTGGCATCC-3′ and reverse 5′-AACATTCCTACCACCAGCAACC-3′ for *PTGS2*; forward 5′-AGCTTCTTTGGGACACTTGC-3′ and reverse 5′-ATAGCAGCCACCTTCATTCC-3′ for *CCL2* and forward 5′-CATACTCCTGCTTGCTGATCC-3′ and reverse 5′-GATGCAGAAGGAGATCACTGC-3′ for *ACTB*.

2.7. Statistical Analysis

Data are shown as the mean ± SEM. Statistical comparisons between two or more groups were conducted using a Welch's *t*-test or the Tukey-Kramer method, respectively, with JMP Pro 14 (SAS Institute Inc., Cary, NC, USA). A *p* value less than 0.05 was defined as statistically significant.

3. Results

3.1. Highest Incidence of SAH in Female Rats with the Bilateral Ovariectomy

In reference to established epidemiological evidence, the risk of SAH is higher in postmenopausal or older females than in males and in females before menopause [3–8], we first examined whether the sex difference in the incidence of SAH could be reproduced or not in a rat model of IAs [9] as in human cases, to escape many uncontrollable confounding factors. Rats were subjected to an IA model and the incidence of IA lesions at the anterior or the posterior communicating artery complex and the onset of SAH due to rupture of IA lesions at each site were examined.

In male rats, 15 among 18 animals (83.3%) developed IAs at the anterior or the posterior communicating artery and 3 of these animals had multiple lesions at both artery complex. SAH occurred in 5 among 18 rats or IA lesions (27.8%) during the observation period of 16 weeks after the induction (Figure 1a–c). In female rats without the bilateral ovariectomy, 9 among 17 animals (52.9%) developed IAs at the anterior or the posterior communicating artery and one of these animals had multiple lesions. SAH occurred in 1 among 17 rats (5.9%) or 10 lesions (10.0%) in total in this group (Figure 1a–c). In female rats with bilateral ovariectomy, 9 among 14 animals (64.3%) developed IAs at the anterior or the posterior communicating artery and 1 of these animals had multiple lesions. SAH occurred in 8 among 14 rats (57.1%) or 10 lesions (80.0%) in total in this group (Figure 1a–c). Although the difference in sex or the implementation of ovariectomy did not influence the development of IAs, the combination of these two factors significantly facilitated the rupture of induced IAs in a rat model. The incidence of SAH per induced IA lesions was thus the highest in female rats with bilateral ovariectomy in spite of the significantly lower systolic blood pressure in female rats than in male rats (Figure 1).

3.2. Exacerbation of the IA Pathology in Female Rats with the Bilateral Ovariectomy

To explore mechanisms underlying the effect of sex difference or the implementation of ovariectomy in female animals on the onset of SAH, the histopathological examinations of induced IA lesions were done. The size of induced IAs was significantly larger in female rats with bilateral ovariectomy than that in other groups (Figure 2a,b). Most IA lesions induced in female animals with bilateral ovariectomy ruptured, resulting in SAH (Figure 1). Intriguingly, the remaining unruptured lesions induced were apparently bigger than the ones induced in female animals without the ovariectomy or in male animals (Figure 2a). Immunohistochemical analyses revealed the accumulation of MPO-positive neutrophils and CD68-positive macrophages in arterial walls of the lesions, even in unruptured IA lesions specifically from female animals with bilateral ovariectomy, similarly to ruptured ones (Figure 2c). Such an accumulation of inflammatory cells was only limited in unruptured IA lesions from male animals or female animals without ovariectomy (Figure 2c). Consistently, expression of pro-inflammatory factor TNF-α, which is related with the pathogenesis [12–14], was higher in unruptured lesions from female animals with bilateral ovariectomy than that in male animals or female animals without ovariectomy (Figure 2d). In addition, expression of TNF-α in unruptured lesions from female animals with bilateral ovariectomy was similar to that in ruptured lesions (Figure 2d). In addition, the presence of vasa vasorum with SMA-positive media, which we identified as a histopathological characteristic of ruptured IA lesions [9], could be detected even in unruptured lesions only from female animals with the bilateral ovariectomy, and not in female animals without ovariectomy or male animals (Figure 2e). The unruptured IA lesion induced in female animals with the bilateral ovariectomy thus resembles ruptured lesions. In other words, the bilateral ovariectomy in female animals promotes events underlying rupture of the lesions.

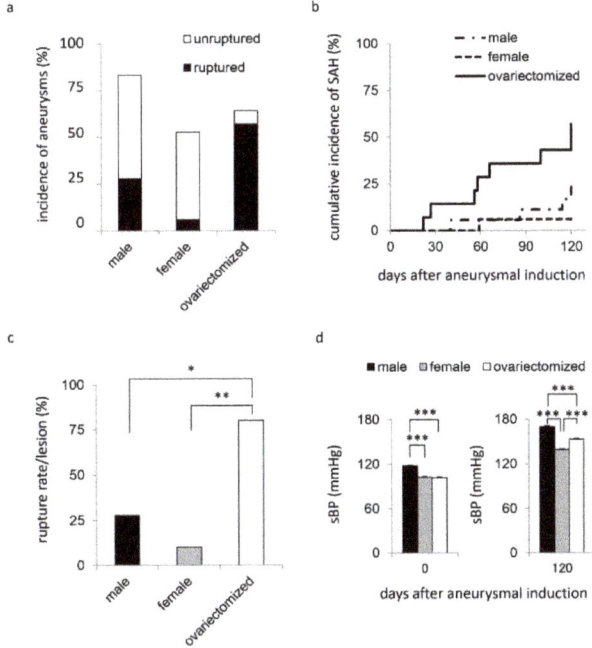

Figure 1. The incidence of intracranial aneurysms, the cumulative incidence of subarachnoid hemorrhage and the rate of rupture of induced lesions. To induce intracranial aneurysms, 10-week-old male (n = 18) or female Sprague–Dawley rats (n = 31) were subjected to the ligation of the left carotid artery, the right external carotid artery and the right pterygopalatine artery, and systemic hypertension by the combination of a high salt diet and the ligation of the left renal artery. In some female rats (n = 14), the bilateral ovariectomy was also applied. Animals were maintained for 120 days after surgical manipulations. The incidence of intracranial aneurysms (**a**), the cumulative incidence of subarachnoid hemorrhage (SAH) (**b**), the rate of rupture of induced lesions (**c**) or systolic blood pressure (sBP) (**d**) in each group; male rats, female rats without ovariectomy (female) or female rats with the bilateral ovariectomy (ovariectomized), are shown. Bars in (**d**) indicate the mean ± SEM. Statistical analysis was done by the Tukey-Kramer method in (**c**,**d**). * $p < 0.05$, ** $p < 0.01$, *** $p < 0.001$.

3.3. Disturbance in Endothelial Function by the Bilateral Ovariectomy in Female Rats

A series of studies about IAs has clarified the involvement of macrophage-mediated chronic inflammatory responses in the pathogenesis of the disease and also the potential contribution of wall shear stress to this process [15–20]. To explore mechanisms regulating ovariectomy-mediated facilitation of rupture of lesions, we examined the effect of the bilateral ovariectomy on endothelial cell function by using the stenosis model of the carotid artery in which the post-stenotic dilatation occurs in response to increased wall shear stress-loading [10,11]. In female rats without ovariectomy, the post-stenotic dilatation of the carotid artery could be observed at 30 min after the partial ligation, as expected (Figure 3a). However, in female animals with the bilateral ovariectomy, the post-stenotic dilatation was partially but significantly restricted (Figure 3a). Importantly, hormone replacement therapy by Estradiol valerate restored ovariectomy-induced restriction of post-stenotic dilatation (Figure 3b). The bilateral ovariectomy thus disturbed endothelial cell function.

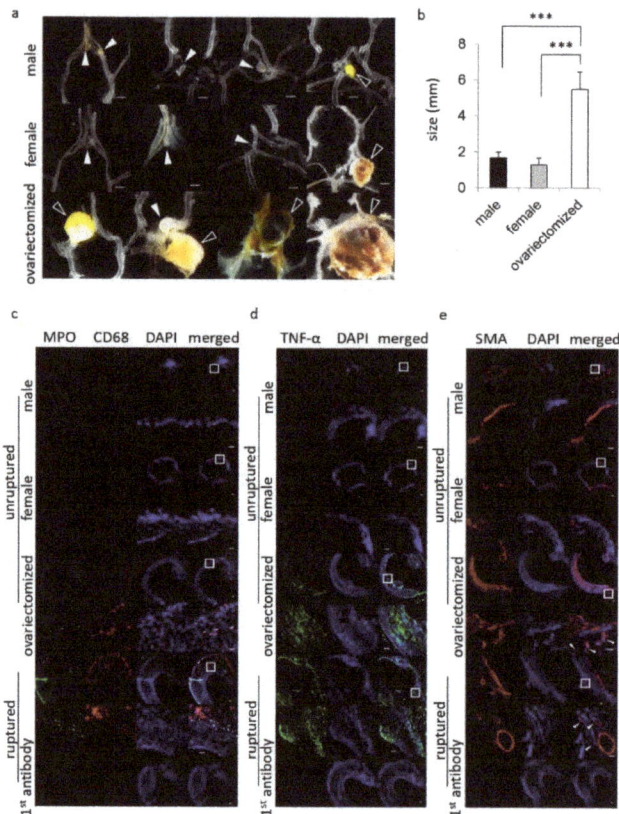

Figure 2. The exacerbation of the pathology of intracranial aneurysm in female rats with the bilateral ovariectomy. Ten-week-old female Sprague–Dawley rats were subjected to the aneurysm model. At 120 days after the surgical manipulations, specimens of induced lesions were harvested. (**a,b**) The macroscopic image of induced lesions (**a**) and their size (**b**) in each group; male rats ($n = 18$), female rats without ovariectomy (female, $n = 10$) or female rats with the bilateral ovariectomy (ovariectomized, $n = 10$). Bar, 1.0 mm (**a**). The white arrows and the black ones in (**a**) indicate the unruptured and the ruptured lesions, respectively. Bars in (**b**) indicate the mean ± SEM. Statistical analysis was done by the Tukey–Kramer method. ***; $p < 0.001$. (**c,d**) show similarity of unruptured lesions induced in female animals with the bilateral ovariectomy with ruptured ones. The representative images of immunostaining for a marker for neutrophil, myeloperoxidase (MPO, green in (**c**)), a marker for macrophage, CD68 (red in (**c**)), TNF-α (green in (**d**)), a marker for smooth muscle cell, smooth muscle alpha-actin (SMA, red in (**e**)), nuclear staining by DAPI (blue) or merged images are shown. The immunostaining without a 1st antibody served as a negative control and the representative images of this staining are shown in the lowest panels. Ruptured lesions were from female rats with the bilateral ovariectomy. The arrow in (**e**) indicates vasa vasorum with SMA-positive media. The magnified images, corresponding to a square in the upper panels, are shown in the lower panels. Bar, 20 μm.

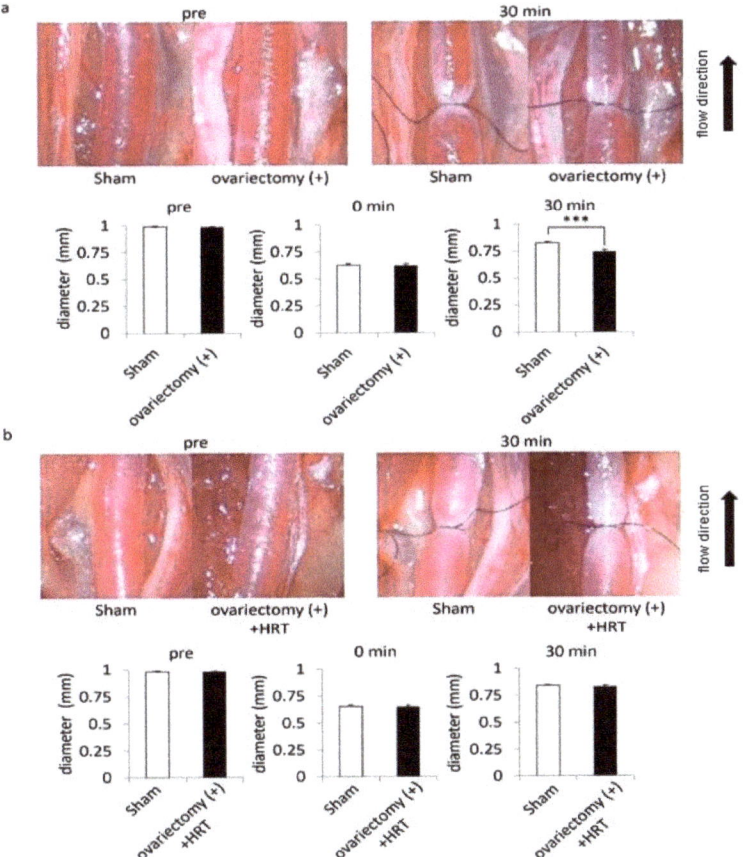

Figure 3. The disturbance of post-stenotic dilatation by the bilateral ovariectomy in female rats. 10-week-old female Sprague–Dawley rats were subjected to the bilateral ovariectomy or a sham-operation. On the 7th day, animals underwent the carotid ligation and the post-stenotic dilatation was observed for following 30 min (**a**). In some animals, hormone replacement therapy (HRT) was applied after the bilateral ovariectomy (**b**). Representative macroscopic images of the carotid artery before (pre) and 30 min after the ligation (30 min) are shown. The diameter of the carotid artery was calculated before (pre), just after (0 min) and 30 min after the ligation (30 min). Bars indicate the mean ± SEM ($n = 4$). Statistical analysis was done by a Welch's t test. ***; $p < 0.001$.

3.4. Suppressive Effect of Sex Hormone on Inflammatory Responses in Macrophages and Neutrophils

Further, we examined the effect of the sex hormone, E2 (the hormone from the ovary) or DHT (the hormone from the testis), on inflammatory responses by cultured macrophages (RAW264.7 cell line) or neutrophils (HL-60 cell line). In RAW264.7 cells, although LPS-induced expressions of pro-inflammatory genes are related with pathogenesis, Tnf (TNF-α) [12–14], Il1b (IL-1β) [21], Ptgs2 (COX-2) [22] or Ccl2 (MCP-1) [20,23]—even with the pre-treatment by E2, the addition of E2 could significantly suppress expressions of all of these genes compared with those in the vehicle-treated cells (Figure 4a). The pre-treatment with DHT significantly suppressed expression of Ccl2 among four genes examined (Figure 4a). In HL-60 cells, the pre-treatment of E2 or DHT suppressed LPS-induced expression of pro-inflammatory genes (Figure 4b) in RAW264.7 cells. The suppressive effect of E2 was stronger than that of DHT as well (Figure 4b). Consistently, expression of TNF-α was higher in lesions from female animals with bilateral ovariectomy than that in male animals or female animals without ovariectomy (Figure 2d). The results of the in vitro study suggest the suppressive effect of the sex hormone on the inflammatory responses in lesions promotes the pathology.

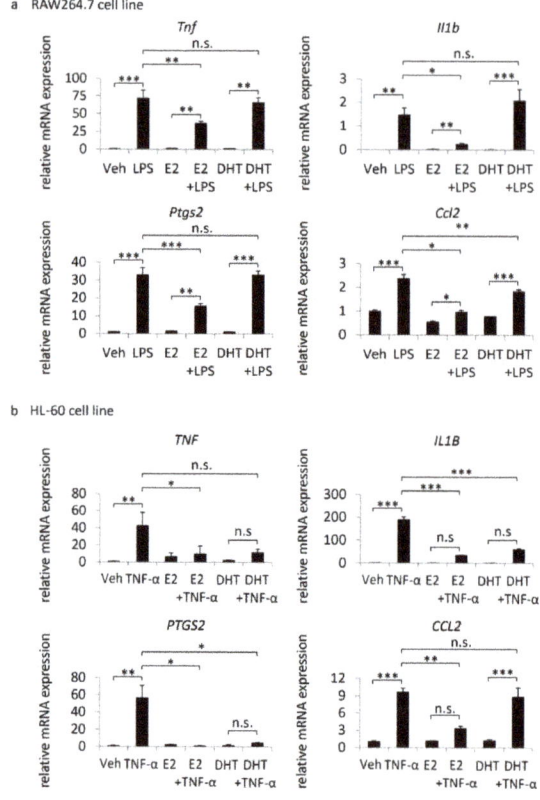

Figure 4. Suppressive effect of the sex hormone on expressions of pro-inflammatory genes in cultured macrophages or neutrophils. RAW264.7 cells (**a**) or HL-60 cells (**b**) were pre-treated with β-estradiol (E2, 50 µg/mL) or 5α-dihydrotestosterone (DHT, 50 µg/mL) for 24 h or 3 h, respectively. Cells were then stimulated with vehicle (Veh), LPS (dose) or TNF-α (dose) for an additional 60 min. Expressions of pro-inflammatory genes were examined by quantitative RT-PCR analyses. Bars indicate the mean ± SEM (n = 4). Statistical analysis was done by a Tukey-Kramer method. *; $p < 0.05$, **; $p < 0.01$, ***; $p < 0.001$. n.s.; statistically not significant.

4. Discussion

The epidemiological findings that post-menopausal females have a higher incidence of IAs than do males or females with menopause [3–8] was reproduced in the rat model in the present study, in which the bilateral ovariectomy in female animals significantly increased rupture of IAs. In another animal model, in which SAH was induced by the combination of the bilateral ovariectomy in female animals with the intrathecal injection of elastase, hormone replacement therapy by estrogen was shown to ameliorate the incidence of rupture [24]. The different animal models of SAH have thus consistently demonstrated the promoting effect of the bilateral ovariectomy on the rupture of IAs, confirming the crucial contribution of estrogen to the rupture of IAs. The previous experimental studies using an animal model of IAs have also demonstrated the facilitation of the formation and the progression of IAs by bilateral ovariectomy, which could be ameliorated by hormone replacement therapy [25,26]. In this report, similar to the present study, the protective role of estrogen in endothelial cell function has been indicated [26]. Furthermore, in human cases, the protective effect of hormone replacement therapy to compensate for the defect in functions of the ovary on the onset of SAH was reported [4,27], suggesting the clinical relevance of the present study. Hormone replacement therapy has adverse effects, such as the increased risk of breast cancer, ischemic stroke and ischemic heart disease, which makes the application of this therapy for the treatment of IAs in post-menopausal women controversial. However, the present study has provided experimental evidence for the potential of hormone replacement therapy as an option of treatment to prevent the onset of SAH in post-menopausal women.

Recent experimental studies mainly using an animal model of IAs [28,29] have clarified the involvement of chronic inflammatory responses in the process regulating the initiation, progression or rupture of IAs [15,16,18,30,31]. Additionally, hemodynamic force, especially wall shear stress, is considered a mediator of IA formation and progression, mainly through a series of studies by computational fluid dynamics analyses [17,32]. In the present study, we clarified the suppressive effect of E2 or DHT on expressions of pro-inflammatory factors in cultured macrophages and neutrophils (Figure 4). Additionally, the combination of female sex with bilateral ovariectomy exacerbated inflammatory cells like macrophages or neutrophils in lesions (Figure 2). Here, the in vitro finding that the suppressive effect of E2 was stronger than that of DHT may be responsible for the highest incidence of rupture in female animals with bilateral ovariectomy. Furthermore, in the stenosis model, the bilateral ovariectomy in female animals disturbed the high wall shear stress-induced post-stenotic dilatation of the carotid artery (Figure 3), suggesting the malfunction of endothelial cells. Intriguingly, the results of the present study have implied the role of the maladaptation of endothelial cells to shear stress-loading at the bifurcation sites as a trigger of molecular events, leading to the progression and rupture of the lesions. The ovariectomy in female animals, therefore, facilitates the pathogenesis of IAs in multiple steps by influencing the functions of endothelial cells and inflammatory cells.

5. Conclusions

To explore mechanisms regulating rupture of IAs, we have used a rat model and revealed the facilitation of the progression or rupture of the lesions by the combination of the female sex and the bilateral ovariectomy. Furthermore, we have clarified the point of actions of sex hormone as endothelial cells and inflammatory cells to inhibit the progression of the pathogenesis. The results of the present study have thus provided new insights about mechanisms regulating the progression of the disease.

Author Contributions: Conceptualization, M.O. and T.A.; data curation, T.A.; formal analysis, M.O.; funding acquisition, T.A.; investigation, M.O., I.O., K.S., M.K., H.M. and T.A.; methodology, M.O., I.O., K.S., M.K. and H.M.; project administration, T.A.; resources, T.A.; software, M.O.; supervision, T.K.; validation, M.O., I.O., K.S., M.K. and H.M.; writing—original draft, M.O. and T.A.; writing—review and editing, T.A. All authors have read and agreed to the published version of the manuscript.

Funding: This research was funded by Core Research for Evolutional Science and Technology (CREST) on Mechanobiology from the Japan Agency for Medical Research and Development (AMED), grant number JP18gm0810006 and JP19gm0810006.

Conflicts of Interest: M.K. was supported by CREST on Mechanobiology from AMED, grant number JP18gm0810006 and JP19gm0810006, until 31 March, 2020. The other authors declare that they have no known competing financial interests or personal relationships that could have appeared to influence the work reported in this paper. The funders had no role in the design of the study; in the collection, analyses, or interpretation of data; in the writing of the manuscript, or in the decision to publish the results.

References

1. Lawton, M.T.; Vates, G.E. Subarachnoid Hemorrhage. *N. Engl. J. Med.* **2017**, *377*, 257–266. [CrossRef] [PubMed]
2. Macdonald, R.L.; Schweizer, T.A. Spontaneous subarachnoid haemorrhage. *Lancet* **2017**, *389*, 655–666. [CrossRef]

3. Yamada, S.; Koizumi, A.; Iso, H.; Wada, Y.; Watanabe, Y.; Date, C.; Yamamoto, A.; Kikuchi, S.; Inaba, Y.; Toyoshima, H.; et al. Risk factors for fatal subarachnoid hemorrhage: The Japan Collaborative Cohort Study. *Stroke* **2003**, *34*, 2781–2787. [CrossRef] [PubMed]
4. Longstreth, W.T.; Nelson, L.M.; Koepsell, T.D.; van Belle, G. Subarachnoid hemorrhage and hormonal factors in women. A population-based case-control study. *Ann. Intern. Med.* **1994**, *121*, 168–173. [CrossRef] [PubMed]
5. Ding, C.; Toll, V.; Ouyang, B.; Chen, M. Younger age of menopause in women with cerebral aneurysms. *J. Neurointerv. Surg.* **2013**, *5*, 327–331. [CrossRef]
6. Horiuchi, T.; Tanaka, Y.; Hongo, K. Sex-related differences in patients treated surgically for aneurysmal subarachnoid hemorrhage. *Neurol. Med. Chir. (Tokyo)* **2006**, *46*, 328–332. [CrossRef]
7. Imaizumi, Y.; Mizutani, T.; Shimizu, K.; Sato, Y.; Taguchi, J. Detection rates and sites of unruptured intracranial aneurysms according to sex and age: An analysis of MR angiography-based brain examinations of 4070 healthy Japanese adults. *J. Neurosurg.* **2018**, *130*, 573–578. [CrossRef]
8. Desai, M.; Wali, A.R.; Birk, H.S.; Santiago-Dieppa, D.R.; Khalessi, A.A. Role of pregnancy and female sex steroids on aneurysm formation, growth, and rupture: A systematic review of the literature. *Neurosurg. Focus* **2019**, *47*, E8. [CrossRef]
9. Miyata, H.; Imai, H.; Koseki, H.; Shimizu, K.; Abekura, Y.; Oka, M.; Kawamata, T.; Matsuda, T.; Nozaki, K.; Narumiya, S.; et al. Vasa vasorum formation is associated with rupture of intracranial aneurysms. *J. Neurosurg.* **2019**. [CrossRef]
10. Cheng, C.; van Haperen, R.; de Waard, M.; van Damme, L.C.; Tempel, D.; Hanemaaijer, L.; van Cappellen, G.W.; Bos, J.; Slager, C.J.; Duncker, D.J.; et al. Shear stress affects the intracellular distribution of eNOS: Direct demonstration by a novel in vivo technique. *Blood* **2005**, *106*, 3691–3698. [CrossRef]
11. Winkel, L.C.; Hoogendoorn, A.; Xing, R.; Wentzel, J.J.; Van der Heiden, K. Animal models of surgically manipulated flow velocities to study shear stress-induced atherosclerosis. *Atherosclerosis* **2015**, *241*, 100–110. [CrossRef] [PubMed]
12. Aoki, T.; Fukuda, M.; Nishimura, M.; Nozaki, K.; Narumiya, S. Critical role of TNF-alpha-TNFR1 signaling in intracranial aneurysm formation. *Acta Neuropathol. Commun.* **2014**, *2*, 34. [CrossRef] [PubMed]
13. Starke, R.M.; Chalouhi, N.; Jabbour, P.M.; Tjoumakaris, S.I.; Gonzalez, L.F.; Rosenwasser, R.H.; Wada, K.; Shimada, K.; Hasan, D.M.; Greig, N.H.; et al. Critical role of TNF-alpha in cerebral aneurysm formation and progression to rupture. *J. Neuroinflamm.* **2014**, *11*, 77. [CrossRef] [PubMed]
14. Yokoi, T.; Isono, T.; Saitoh, M.; Yoshimura, Y.; Nozaki, K. Suppression of cerebral aneurysm formation in rats by a tumor necrosis factor-alpha inhibitor. *J. Neurosurg.* **2014**, *120*, 1193–1200. [CrossRef]
15. Shimizu, K.; Kushamae, M.; Mizutani, T.; Aoki, T. Intracranial Aneurysm as a Macrophage-mediated Inflammatory Disease. *Neurol. Med. Chir. (Tokyo)* **2019**, *59*, 126–132. [CrossRef] [PubMed]
16. Fukuda, M.; Aoki, T. Molecular basis for intracranial aneurysm formation. *Acta Neurochir. Suppl.* **2015**, *120*, 13–15.
17. Frosen, J.; Cebral, J.; Robertson, A.M.; Aoki, T. Flow-induced, inflammation-mediated arterial wall remodeling in the formation and progression of intracranial aneurysms. *Neurosurg. Focus* **2019**, *47*, E21. [CrossRef]
18. Aoki, T.; Frosen, J.; Fukuda, M.; Bando, K.; Shioi, G.; Tsuji, K.; Ollikainen, E.; Nozaki, K.; Laakkonen, J.; Narumiya, S. Prostaglandin E2-EP2-NF-kappaB signaling in macrophages as a potential therapeutic target for intracranial aneurysms. *Sci. Signal* **2017**, *10*. [CrossRef]
19. Aoki, T.; Kataoka, H.; Shimamura, M.; Nakagami, H.; Wakayama, K.; Moriwaki, T.; Ishibashi, R.; Nozaki, K.; Morishita, R.; Hashimoto, N. NF-kappaB is a key mediator of cerebral aneurysm formation. *Circulation* **2007**, *116*, 2830–2840. [CrossRef]
20. Aoki, T.; Kataoka, H.; Ishibashi, R.; Nozaki, K.; Egashira, K.; Hashimoto, N. Impact of monocyte chemoattractant protein-1 deficiency on cerebral aneurysm formation. *Stroke* **2009**, *40*, 942–951. [CrossRef]
21. Moriwaki, T.; Takagi, Y.; Sadamasa, N.; Aoki, T.; Nozaki, K.; Hashimoto, N. Impaired progression of cerebral aneurysms in interleukin-1beta-deficient mice. *Stroke* **2006**, *37*, 900–905. [CrossRef] [PubMed]
22. Aoki, T.; Nishimura, M.; Matsuoka, T.; Yamamoto, K.; Furuyashiki, T.; Kataoka, H.; Kitaoka, S.; Ishibashi, R.; Ishibazawa, A.; Miyamoto, S.; et al. PGE(2) -EP(2) signalling in endothelium is activated by haemodynamic stress and induces cerebral aneurysm through an amplifying loop via NF-kappaB. *Br. J. Pharm.* **2011**, *163*, 1237–1249. [CrossRef] [PubMed]

23. Kanematsu, Y.; Kanematsu, M.; Kurihara, C.; Tada, Y.; Tsou, T.L.; van Rooijen, N.; Lawton, M.T.; Young, W.L.; Liang, E.I.; Nuki, Y.; et al. Critical roles of macrophages in the formation of intracranial aneurysm. *Stroke* **2011**, *42*, 173–178. [CrossRef] [PubMed]
24. Tada, Y.; Wada, K.; Shimada, K.; Makino, H.; Liang, E.I.; Murakami, S.; Kudo, M.; Shikata, F.; Pena Silva, R.A.; Kitazato, K.T.; et al. Estrogen protects against intracranial aneurysm rupture in ovariectomized mice. *Hypertension* **2014**, *63*, 1339–1344. [CrossRef] [PubMed]
25. Jamous, M.A.; Nagahiro, S.; Kitazato, K.T.; Satomi, J.; Satoh, K. Role of estrogen deficiency in the formation and progression of cerebral aneurysms. Part I: Experimental study of the effect of oophorectomy in rats. *J. Neurosurg.* **2005**, *103*, 1046–1051. [CrossRef] [PubMed]
26. Jamous, M.A.; Nagahiro, S.; Kitazato, K.T.; Tamura, T.; Kuwayama, K.; Satoh, K. Role of estrogen deficiency in the formation and progression of cerebral aneurysms. Part II: Experimental study of the effects of hormone replacement therapy in rats. *J. Neurosurg.* **2005**, *103*, 1052–1057. [CrossRef]
27. Mhurchu, C.N.; Anderson, C.; Jamrozik, K.; Hankey, G.; Dunbabin, D.; Australasian Cooperative Research on Subarachnoid Hemorrhage Study (ACROSS) Group. Hormonal factors and risk of aneurysmal subarachnoid hemorrhage: An international population-based, case-control study. *Stroke* **2001**, *32*, 606–612. [CrossRef]
28. Aoki, T.; Miyata, H.; Abekura, Y.; Koseki, H.; Shimizu, K. Rat Model of Intracranial Aneurysm: Variations, Usefulness, and Limitations of the Hashimoto Model. *Acta Neurochir. Suppl.* **2020**, *127*, 35–41.
29. Strange, F.; Gruter, B.E.; Fandino, J.; Marbacher, S. Preclinical Intracranial Aneurysm Models: A Systematic Review. *Brain Sci.* **2020**, *10*, 134. [CrossRef]
30. Aoki, T.; Narumiya, S. Prostaglandins and chronic inflammation. *Trends Pharm. Sci.* **2012**, *33*, 304–311. [CrossRef]
31. Tulamo, R.; Frosen, J.; Hernesniemi, J.; Niemela, M. Inflammatory changes in the aneurysm wall: A review. *J. Neurointerv. Surg.* **2018**, *10*, i58–i67. [CrossRef] [PubMed]
32. Diagbouga, M.R.; Morel, S.; Bijlenga, P.; Kwak, B.R. Role of hemodynamics in initiation/growth of intracranial aneurysms. *Eur. J. Clin. Investig.* **2018**, *48*, e12992. [CrossRef] [PubMed]

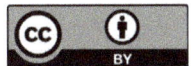

© 2020 by the authors. Licensee MDPI, Basel, Switzerland. This article is an open access article distributed under the terms and conditions of the Creative Commons Attribution (CC BY) license (http://creativecommons.org/licenses/by/4.0/).

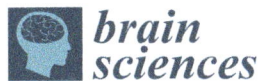

Article

Endovascular Temporary Balloon Occlusion for Microsurgical Clipping of Posterior Circulation Aneurysms

Jenny C. Kienzler [1], Michael Diepers [2], Serge Marbacher [1], Luca Remonda [2] and Javier Fandino [1,*]

1. Department of Neurosurgery, Kantonsspital Aarau, CH-5000 Aarau, Switzerland; jenny.kienzler@ksa.ch (J.C.K.); serge.Marbacher@ksa.ch (S.M.)
2. Division of Neuroradiology, Department of Radiology, Kantonsspital Aarau, 5000 Aarau, Switzerland; michael.diepers@ksa.ch (M.D.); luca.remonda@ksa.ch (L.R.)
* Correspondence: fandino@neurochirurgie-ag.ch; Tel.: +41-62-838-6692; Fax: +41-62-838-6629

Received: 5 April 2020; Accepted: 27 May 2020; Published: 30 May 2020

Abstract: Based on the relationship between the posterior clinoid process and the basilar artery (BA) apex it may be difficult to obtain proximal control of the BA using temporary clips. Endovascular BA temporary balloon occlusion (TBO) can reduce aneurysm sac pressure, facilitate dissection/clipping, and finally lower the risk of intraoperative rupture. We present our experience with TBO during aneurysm clipping of posterior circulation aneurysms within the setting of a hybrid operating room (hOR). We report one case each of a basilar tip, posterior cerebral artery, and superior cerebellar artery aneurysm that underwent surgical occlusion under TBO within an hOR. Surgical exposure of the BA was achieved with a pterional approach and selective anterior and posterior clinoidectomy. Intraoperative digital subtraction angiography (iDSA) was performed prior, during, and after aneurysm occlusion. Two patients presented with subarachnoid hemorrhage and one patient presented with an unruptured aneurysm. The intraluminal balloon was inserted through the femoral artery and inflated in the BA after craniotomy to allow further dissection of the parent vessel and branches needed for the preparation of the aneurysm neck. No complications during balloon inflation and aneurysm dissection occurred. Intraoperative aneurysm rupture prior to clipping did not occur. The duration of TBO varied between 9 and 11 min. Small neck aneurysm remnants were present in two cases (BA and PCA). Two patients recovered well with a GOS 5 after surgery and one patient died due to complications unrelated to surgery. Intraoperative TBO within the hOR is a feasible and safe procedure with no additional morbidity when using a standardized protocol and setting. No relevant side effects or intraoperative complications were present in this series. In addition, iDSA in an hOR facilitates the evaluation of the surgical result and 3D reconstructions provide documentation of potential aneurysm remnants for future follow-up.

Keywords: aneurysm clipping; posterior circulation aneurysm; temporary balloon occlusion; intraoperative digital subtraction angiography; hybrid operating room

1. Introduction

Aneurysms of the posterior circulation, such as the basilar artery (BA), present a particular surgical challenge [1,2]. They represent 5–8% of all intracranial aneurysms and more than 50% of those in the posterior circulation [3,4]. Posterior circulation aneurysms are known to have a higher risk of rupture [5]. According to recently published scores such as PHASES [6] or UIATS [7], preventive endovascular or surgical methods can be performed in patients at risk, to minimize the chance of aneurysm rupture. The difficulties of microsurgical clipping are mainly caused by anatomical conditions and a demanding approach [8]. Surgical complexity varies according to size, shape, and localization of the aneurysm, degree of intraoperative brain swelling, and the microsurgical experience of the surgeon [9]. Moreover, standard clipping could fail due to insufficient proximal control and lead to incomplete occlusion or intraoperative aneurysm rupture [10]. Nevertheless, microsurgical clipping is still more accessible worldwide, especially in developing countries [11].

The ISAT (International Subarachnoid Aneurysm Trial) reported a higher rupture rate for basilar apex aneurysm in correlation with aneurysm size [12]. Increased morbidity and mortality, and worse clinical outcome was also reported after surgical clipping compared to endovascular coiling of a posterior circulation aneurysm [12]. These findings initiated the use of endovascular treatment for a basilar apex region aneurysm [13]. The fact that fewer neurosurgeons are performing microsurgical clipping of basilar apex aneurysm supports the trend for treating basilar artery aneurysms endovascularly rather than surgically [14]. The safety of endovascular occlusion of BA aneurysms has been proven, although long-term sustainability and efficacy remain unclear [13–17].

Up to 50% recanalization and regrowth of a coiled aneurysm has been reported [17–20]. The annual risk of bleeding in a partially coiled or recanalized aneurysm is reported to range from 2.1–15% [17,18,21–23]. This is relatively high and similar to rates for an unruptured aneurysm [5,24–29].

The exact location of the aneurysm is the key factor when deciding which surgical approach to take. The prevention of any injury to the brainstem and its perforators is crucial [30]. Different approaches to BA aneurysms have been described including the pterional approach introduced by G. Yasargil [31], the subtemporal approach pioneered by C. Drake [32], as well as lateral supraorbital [33], orbitozygomatic [34,35], modified presigmoid [36], transpetrosal [37] or transzygomatic transcavernous approaches, [13] and many others [38,39].

Various methods of temporary vessel occlusion or local blood flow interruption have been applied to facilitate a microsurgical approach to a large aneurysm in a narrow and deep location. Also, adenosine-induced cardiac arrest [40], hypothermic circulatory arrest [41], temporary clip placement [42], and temporary balloon occlusion [43] have been described. The relationship between the posterior clinoid process and the BA apex may limit the access for temporary clips [39]. An endovascular technique using balloon inflation in the parent vessel of the aneurysm can achieve proximal and distal control during surgery and, therefore, eliminate the need for temporary clipping [43]. Intraoperative temporary balloon occlusion (TBO) of the parent vessel might lower the risk of intraoperative rupture, reduce pressure in the aneurysm sac, and facilitate dissection and microsurgical clipping. The aim of this study is to describe the technical issues, setup, and experience of intraoperative TBO during surgical occlusion of complex posterior circulation aneurysms within the hybrid operating room (hOR).

2. Materials and Methods

We report three cases of intracranial aneurysms of the posterior circulation that underwent clipping with the concurrent use of TBO in our department between 2013 and 2016. The first patient suffered subarachnoid hemorrhage (SAH) after the rupture of a basilar tip aneurysm (16 × 16 × 15 mm). Endovascular occlusion was not indicated due to the risk of occlusion of the posterior cerebral artery (PCA) and the superior cerebellar artery (SCA). The second case presented with a ruptured, partially thrombosed BA aneurysm (11 × 8 × 8 mm) with secondary wall hematoma and no SAH. As in the previous case, endovascular occlusion was considered not possible due to the risk of SCA occlusion caused by duplicate origin from the aneurysm fundus. The third patient had an incidental right proximal PCA (P1) aneurysm (4 × 5 × 5 mm). Endovascular treatment was scheduled, but 3D digital cerebral angiography (DSA) showed the SCA originating from the aneurysm sac and the treatment strategy was changed to surgery occlusion. Complex anatomical vascular findings were considered for the decision to choose a combined endovascular and microsurgical procedure within the (hOR) in these three cases (Table 1).

Table 1. Demographic characteristics, clinical findings, aneurysm description, and outcome parameters.

Case	Age (Years)	Gender	Aneurysm Location and Anatomical Variation	Aneurysm Size (mm)	Previous Treatment	Clinical Presentation	Fisher Grade	H and H/WFNS Grade	GCS	mRS	GOS
1	53	Female	Basilar tip aneurysm Bilateral PCA and SCA are leaving from the aneurysm base	16 × 16 × 15	no	Dizziness attack and syncope, SAH	4	5/5	3	6	1
2	44	Male	Partially thrombosed distal left side dissecting basilar artery aneurysm with secondary wall hematoma Ampullary exit of the left double-laid SCA from the aneurysm fundus	11 × 8 × 8	no	Thunderclap headache	N/A	N/A	15	0	5
3	48	Female	Proximal right side PCA aneurysm (P1 branch) Right SCA exits the P1 segment from the aneurysms side wall	4 × 5 × 5	no	Incidental finding Diagnostic in the context of a vestibular syndrome	N/A	N/A	15	0	5

PCA = posterior cerebral artery, SCA = superior cerebellar artery, SAH = subarachnoid hemorrhage, N/A = not available, H and H = Hunt and Hess, GCS = Glasgow Comma Scale, mRS = modified Rankin Scale, GOS = Glasgow Outcome Scale.

The technical aspects of performed combined approaches in the hOR have been described by our group in an earlier publication [44]. The main unit consists of a 360° radiolucent carbon fiber table (Alphamaquet 1150, Maquet AG, Switzerland) that is coupled with the C-arm angiography system (Allura Xper FD20, Philips, Netherlands). A radiolucent head holder and pins are required for optimal acquisition of angiograms and intraoperative CT scans (Mayfield, Integra GmbH, Ratingen, Germany). A 7-Fr sheath is placed in the right or left femoral artery in preparation for intraoperative endovascular balloon occlusion and control DSA. All cases underwent an intraoperative DSA (iDSA) and CT (iCT) scan before they were transferred to the intensive care unit.

2.1. Illustrative Cases

The surgical approach and endovascular techniques were similar in all three cases.

2.1.1. Surgical Procedure

After the positioning of the patient's head in a carbon clamp in the hOR, a right fronto-temporal craniotomy and selective extradural anterior clinoidectomy were performed. The proximal Sylvian fissure was opened, and the chiasmatic cistern incised, followed by dissection of the optic and oculomotor nerve, and carotid artery. Once the posterior clinoid process was exposed, a posterior clinoidectomy was completed with a 2 mm drill. The afterward visible BA, PCA's, SCA's, and aneurysm were inspected. After craniotomy, the first iDSA was performed by cannulation of the right femoral artery with a 7-Fr sheath and inserting a 5F diagnostic catheter in one of the vertebral arteries. The first iDSA showed the previously identified aneurysm and in Case 1 a progression of the dissecting basilar tip aneurysm with a new bleb. The diagnostic catheter was exchanged for a soft guiding catheter (Neuron 6F 058, Penumbra, Alameda CA, USA). An ASCENT® 4 × 7 balloon (DePuy Synthes) and was then placed in the middle or distal segment of the BA and inflated under fluoroscopy to interrupt blood flow. The dual lumen design of the ASCENT balloon allows the distal flushing of the occluded vessel by saline. In the meantime, the BA or PCA aneurysm neck, which was significantly softened, as well as PCA and SCA branches were further dissected. The aneurysms were occluded in a microtechnical fashion with straight standard titanium 790-Yasargil-Clips (Aesculap, Tübingen, Germany) under visualization of both SCA branches. The balloon was deflated after 9, 10, and 11 min of TBO. An iDSA and intraoperative 3D-angiography in Case 1 showed complete occlusion of the BA aneurysm with patent PCA and SCA branches (Figure 1). The iDSA in Cases 2 and 3, revealed a small remnant at the aneurysm neck to preserve the SCA exit, no sign of aneurysm perfusion, and patent PCA and SCA branches (Figures 2 and 3). The dura was sutured, the bone flap fixed, and the wound sutured using a standard multilayered technique. The iCT scan documented no hemorrhage or midline shift.

Case 1

History

This 53-year-old patient presented with a SAH after a sudden loss of consciousness at home. The patient was intubated upon admission with a Glasgow Coma Scale (GCS) score of 3. The CT scan showed a SAH caused by a ruptured basilar tip aneurysm (Fisher grade IV). A DSA was performed after the patient improved to a GCS of 10 following two days of conservative treatment and CSF drainage after ventriculostomy. A basilar tip aneurysm (16 × 16 × 15 mm) with the PCA and SCA bilaterally arising from the aneurysm base was identified. Indication for surgical occlusion was decided after interdisciplinary case discussion. The surgical procedure in the hOR had to be postponed for six days due to severe vasospasms in the posterior circulation.

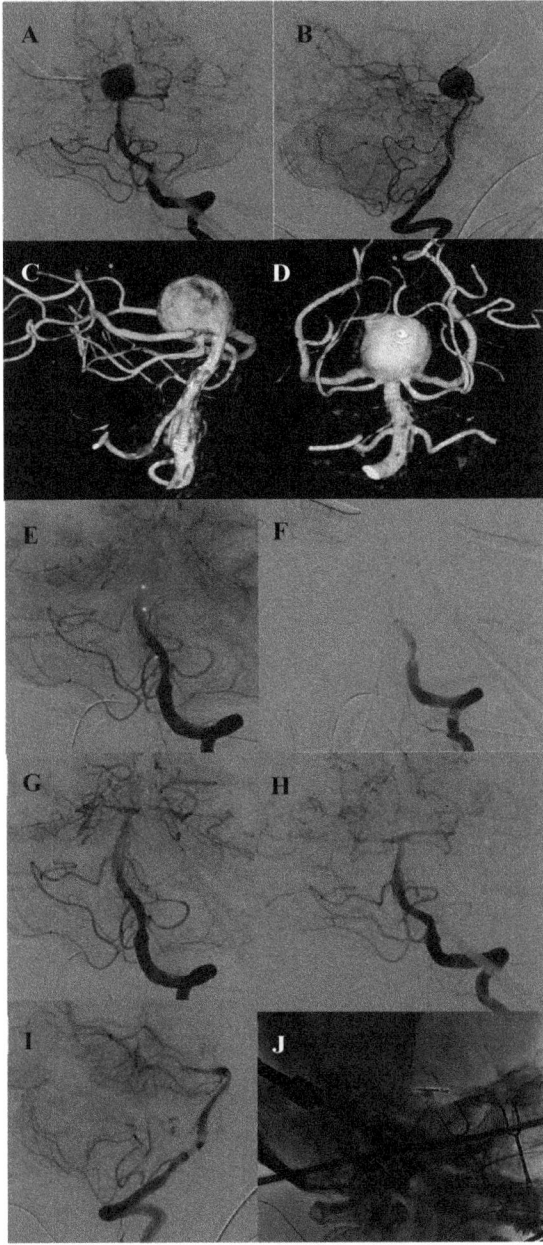

Figure 1. Case 1. Preoperative ap and lateral DSA of the basilar tip aneurysm (**A,B**). Preoperative 3D angiography of the basilar aneurysm presenting the bilateral origin of the PCA and SCA from the aneurysm base (**C,D**). Intraoperative angiography showing the endovascular placement of the balloon and occlusion of the basilar artery (**E,F**). Intraoperative DSA after clipping and closure of the balloon showing complete occlusion of the aneurysm in ap and lateral view with all branches open (**G–I**). Intraoperative picture of the opened skull, placed fish hooks, spatula and clip (**J**).

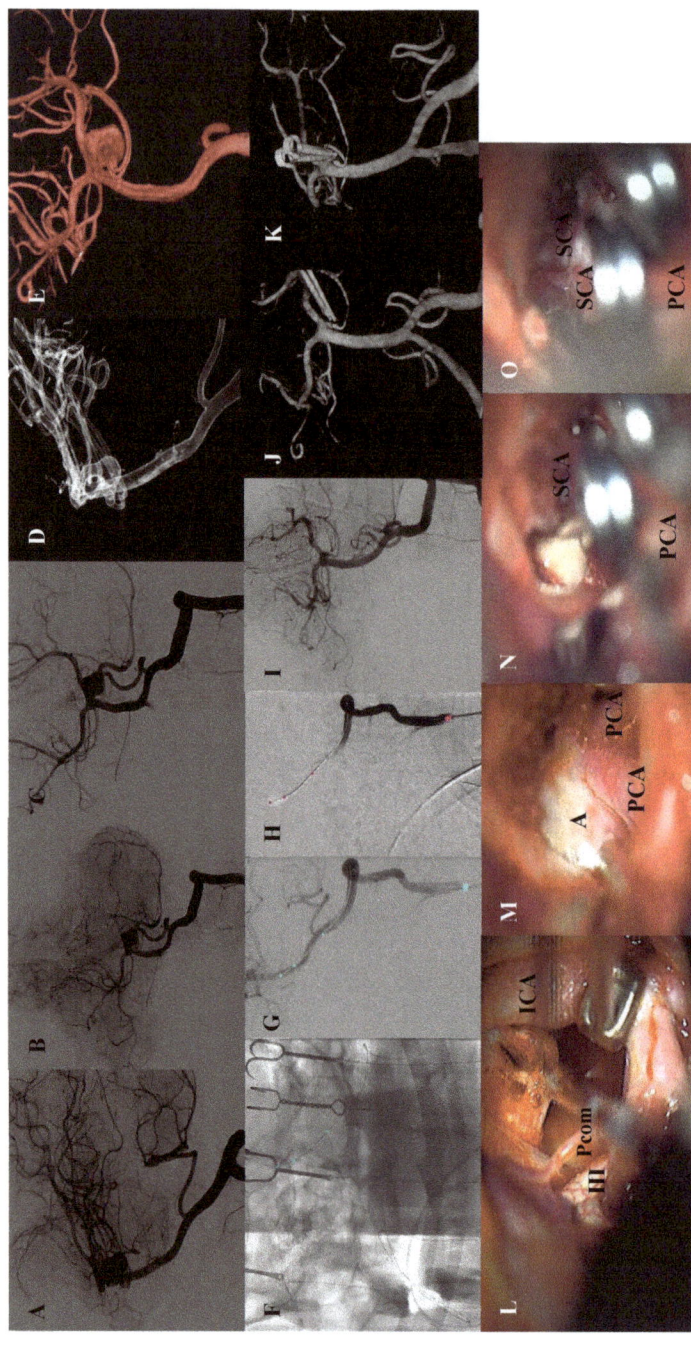

Figure 2. Case 2. Preoperative DSA ap and lateral projections of the left side dissecting basilar artery aneurysm (**A–C**). Preoperative 3D-DSA of the basilar aneurysm, presenting the ampullary exit of the left double-laid SCA from the aneurysm fundus (**D,E**). Intraoperative DSA showing the endovascular placement of the balloon and occlusion of the basilar artery through balloon inflation (**F,G**). Intraoperative angiography after clipping and deflation of the balloon demonstrating occlusion of the aneurysm in the ap and lateral view (**H,I**). Intraoperative 3D angiography in the ap and lateral view, showing a small remnant at the neck of the aneurysm to preserve the SCA exit (**J**). Microsurgical view showing the aneurysm approach with mobilization of the ICA with hook retractor (**K**), BA aneurysm (**L**), and situs after clipping with patency of all branches and parent vessel (**M–O**). Abbreviations: DSA = digital subtraction angiography, SCA = superior cerebellar artery, ICA = internal carotid artery, BA= basilar artery, III = oculomotor nerve, PCA = posterior cerebral artery, A = aneurysm, Pcom = posterior communicating artery.

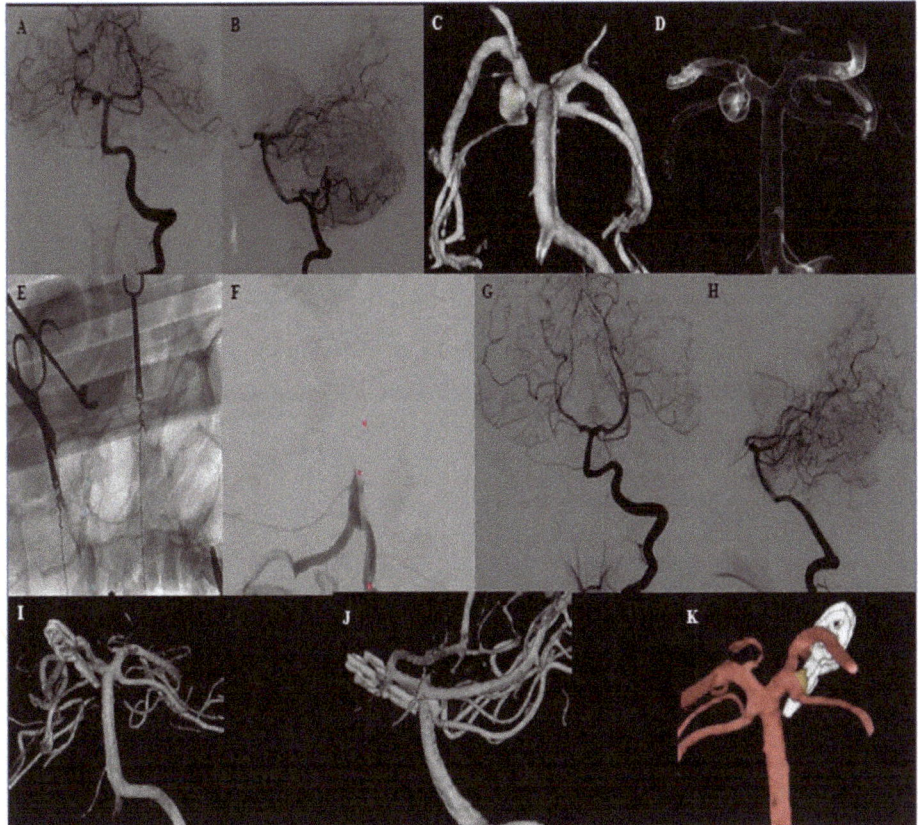

Figure 3. Case 3. Preoperative DSA ap and lateral projections of the proximal right side PCA aneurysm (P1 branch) (**A,B**). Preoperative 3D-DSA of the PCA aneurysm, showing the right SCA leaving the P1 segment from the aneurysm sidewall (**C,D**). Intraoperative DSA presenting the placement of the balloon and occlusion of the BA after balloon inflation (**E,F**). Intraoperative angiography after clipping and balloon removal demonstrating occlusion of the aneurysm and patency of the BA and PCA (**G–I**). Intraoperative 3D-DSA showing a small remnant at the aneurysm neck to preserve the patency of the SCA (**J,K**). Abbreviations: DSA = digital subtraction angiography, PCA = posterior cerebral artery, SCA = superior cerebellar artery.

Postoperative Course

Further course on the ICU was unsuccessful. Consciousness persisted at a low level of GCS 5 due to severe vasospasm and the deterioration of cerebral perfusion on CT was observed within 48 h after surgery. Despite of endovascular spasmolysis with Nimodipine was performed no clinical improvement could be observed. During the next days, the general condition of the patient deteriorated due to pneumonia and respiratory failure leading to death eight days after surgery.

Case 2

History

A 44-year-old patient was admitted to the emergency room with a thunderclap headache, neck pain, vomiting, and paresthesia in the right arm. The patient had a GCS score of 15 without meningism or any neurological deficits. Further investigations (CT, CTA, and DSA) excluded an SAH but showed a dissecting, partially thrombosed BA aneurysm (11 × 8 × 8 mm) with a secondary wall hematoma. Cerebral angiography revealed a duplicate origin of the SCA out of the aneurysm fundus. Treatment options were discussed in the interdisciplinary neurovascular board. In principal, endovascular occlusion by coiling or stent-assisted coiling was considered—with a high risk of SCA occlusion and secondary cerebellar ischemia. Therefore, the group decided to recommend microsurgical aneurysm clipping under endovascular TBO in the hOR.

Postoperative Course

The patient was hospitalized for one more week. During this time, the patient suffered an epileptic seizure. Apart from this, the patient could be rapidly mobilized with a GCS score of 15 and no new neurological deficits.

Case 3

History

After the occurrence of vertigo, this 48-year-old patient underwent an MRI scan which revealed an incidental right PCA aneurysm. The patient was referred to our Institution, and the history and clinical examination excluded any episodes of headache, epileptic seizure, or neurological deficits. Further aneurysm imaging with DSA showed a saccular right BA aneurysm at the origin of the P1 segment of the PCA (4 × 5 × 5 mm). The pre-interventional 3D-DSA depicted the origin of the SCA directly arising from the aneurysm fundus, as well as a hypoplastic bilateral posterior communicating artery. After the case discussion with the neurovascular board, surgical occlusion with TBO in the hOR was recommended.

Postoperative Course

Postoperatively, the patient presented with a GCS score of 15, discrete ptosis, anisocoria, and double vision. A further CT scan confirmed otherwise regular findings (the ophthalmological symptoms were mainly caused by an impairment of oculomotor nerve function). The oculomotor nerve dysfunction had resolved by itself by the three-month follow up.

3. Results

All cases underwent combined surgical and endovascular procedures in our hOR. After craniotomy and dissection of the parent vessel and aneurysm the intraluminal balloon was inserted through the femoral artery and inflated in the BA. In all three cases, intraoperative TBO was successfully performed without complications. No aneurysm rupture prior to clipping, or any other intra- or postoperative problems (necessary clip repositioning, parent vessel or branch occlusion, thromboembolic event, or re-bleeding) occurred. The mean duration of TBO was 10 min (Table 2). Upon inflation of the balloon, the intraluminal pressure releases and the aneurysm softens rapidly, which gives the surgeon more space and flexibility to explore the aneurysm and vessels branching out of the aneurysm base. Intraoperative DSA following clipping confirmed complete aneurysm occlusion with patent parent and branch vessels. In two cases, a small remnant at the aneurysm neck was visible in the intraoperative 3D angiography, which was necessary to preserve the branch origin. Two patients showed good postoperative recovery with GOS 5 and one patient died due to severe vasospasm and pneumonia.

Table 2. Details of the intraoperative balloon occlusion procedure, clipping, and iDSA findings.

Case	Duration of TBO (Min)	Number of Clips	Intraoperative DSA Findings	Balloon Catheter Used	Complications
1	9	1	Complete occlusion of the aneurysm All branches open	ASCENT® 4 × 7 balloon (DePuy Synthes)	None
2	10	2	Small remnant at the neck to preserve the SCA exit No aneurysm perfusion All branches open	ASCENT® 4 × 7 balloon (DePuy Synthes)	None
3	11	3	Small remnant at the neck to preserve the SCA exit No aneurysm perfusion All branches open	ASCENT® 4 × 7 balloon (DePuy Synthes)	None

iDSA = intraoperative digital subtraction angiography, TBO = temporary balloon occlusion, SCA = superior cerebellar artery.

4. Discussion

The findings of this technical note support the fact that TBO is a feasible, safe, and reliable method for the clipping of posterior aneurysms that are technically demanding and complex due to size or anatomy. In our institution, TBO with a combined endovascular and surgical approach is also used for giant and complex recurrent middle cerebral artery (MCA) or anterior communicating artery aneurysms. In cases with a ruptured MCA aneurysm and surrounding hematoma, endovascular TBO facilitated clipping following hematoma evacuation and prevented an intraoperative rupture of fragile high-risk aneurysms.

In the case of intraoperative rupture, TBO could effectively control acute bleeding and increase the safety and accuracy of clip placement. In one case report with the intraoperative rupture of a paraclinoid aneurysm, TBO provided a salvage procedure for adequate hemostasis with additional intraluminal support to preserve the parent artery during clip placement [43].

In our opinion, microsurgery should still be viewed as a valuable option in the management of posterior circulation aneurysms. Various authors have reported good radiological and clinical outcomes for BA clipping with or without additional bypass [33,45–51]. Overall, the most common complications in this location are perforator and branch ischemia-related events and cranial nerve deficits, often involving oculomotor nerve palsies [47,52–54]. One case of transient oculomotor nerve palsy occurred in our series.

The angiographic obliteration rate of posterior circulation aneurysm has been reported with a range from 91.9–98.1% [8,29,45,55]. However, other reports also cited 11.5% transient and 7.8% permanent neurological deteriorations [45].

Circumferential exposure of the aneurysm, including branches and perforators, is necessary prior to a safe and efficacious clip application. Dissection and visualization of where they exit the aneurysm can be very demanding. Various methods have been described to support the surgeon during the clip application. Additional endovascular assistance can help prospective vascular neurosurgeons to become more confident and proficient in these cases. Temporary parent vessel occlusion seems to be a safe procedure. Interestingly, a study with a mean follow-up of 53 months showed that a temporary artery occlusion time (mean 16.1 min) had no effect on overall long-term clinical outcomes [56].

The "gold standard" for proximal vessel control is a temporary clip application, which is not always feasible, especially in areas with limited access [57]. Proximal parent vessel ligation [58] can be considered for treating giant aneurysms. Transient asystole with adenosine [40,59,60], deep hypothermic circulatory arrest [61], or rapid ventricular pacing [62] are other techniques also described in the literature but have higher risk profiles for side effects such as atrial or ventricular fibrillation, arrhythmias, and prolonged hypotension [62]. In addition, the risk of stroke can increase after a circulatory arrest, and the resulting need for a multidisciplinary team of surgeons and technologists is logistically challenging and expensive [63]. Perioperative morbidity and mortality for circulatory arrest has been described as ranging from 8.3–17% [41,61]. The risk of side effects of these different techniques has to be weighed against the significant chance of intraoperative aneurysm rupture, incomplete clipping, or unintended branch occlusion due to poor visualization.

In comparison, TBO presents a simple, fast, and inexpensive technique with no need for special anesthesiological monitoring or training and can be performed at any time in every center with endovascular expertise. Although temporary clipping will remain the routinely used technique, TBO may be more accurate for complex and large aneurysms, especially in the posterior circulation and to prevent premature rupture. In posterior circulation aneurysm clipping, proximal control with temporary clipping is often not possible due to the complex anatomy, skull base proximity, and location near the brain stem and cranial nerves [64]. The temporary clip itself may hinder the placement of the permanent one due to the limited surgical corridor [65]. In these cases, TBO can provide a reliable alternative. Proximal control with TBO can be achieved before craniotomy with minimal obstruction of the surgical field and less brain retraction.

Possible side effects of TBO and temporary clipping include wall injury of the parent vessel or thromboembolic events causing postoperative ischemic deficits. MacDonald et al. compared the degree of acute endothelial injury after temporary vessel occlusion with external clipping and endovascular balloon occlusion in a pig model [66]. The results revealed that vessel injury worsened with time and was more prevalent adjacent to the clip; as compared to the widespread pattern with TBO [66]. There is the concern of a higher risk of ischemic complications with balloon occlusion in perforator-rich vessels like MCA and BA, but neither MCA nor BA TBO interventions at our institution led to perforator infarctions.

The TBO technique was first described in 1986 by Kinjo et al. [67], by Shucart et al. in 1990 [68], and in many other case series since then. More recently, another group has reported on the use of TBO in the hybrid OR [69]. Table 3 provides an overview of the literature to-date.

Most series included large or giant paraclinoid ICA aneurysms occluded with clip ligation after balloon catheter placement in the ICA [69–71]. Intra-luminal pressure was decreased through the additional placement of a temporary clip distal to the aneurysm on the posterior communicating artery to reduce collateral blood flow, as well as the application of the retrograde decompression-suction method in the ICA [69,71,72]. In these series, endovascular TBO eliminated the need for cervical ICA dissection [68,69]. A review of the literature found a total of 188 aneurysms clipped with TBO. The largest series, published by Fulkerson et al [73]. included 63 ophthalmic artery aneurysms. The description of TBO in posterior circulation aneurysms, however, is less common with a total of only 20 cases. Bailes et al. published the first series of TBO use in multiple basilar artery aneurysms [74]. Apart from the recent study, eight other series have used TBO only for successful clipping [64,65,68,70,74–77]. Balloon placement in the aneurysm orifice or neck has only been described in two case series [65,77] and was otherwise performed in the proximal parent vessel. TBO duration ranged from 1.5–3 min for each balloon inflation and a total maximum of 50 min [43,63–65,68,71,75,77–81].

The overall reported complication rate for TBO is very low at 1.7–3.7% [72]. TBO procedure-related thromboembolic events occurred in five patients (2.6%). This risk is increased in cases with pronounced vessel wall sclerosis or prolonged temporary occlusion. One intraoperative balloon rupture and balloon exchange led to a thrombus in the M1 segment, with subsequent intraoperative embolectomy and postoperative transient hemiparesis. Symptoms such as dysphasia and hemiparesis were transient in all other cases except one major MCA infarct, which lead to the death of the patient [71,80–82]. Further TBO-related complications included: ICA intima dissection with ICA occlusion at the neck requiring medical treatment only (recovery was complete after four days) [81], as well as increases in vasospasms due to mechanical wall stimulation with transient hemiparesis [77].

Table 3. Overview of all aneurysm cases including clipping with TBO in the literature. Information includes aneurysm characteristics, TBO duration, additional techniques, aneurysm occlusion status and complications. All posterior circulation aneurysms and complications related to TBO are listed in bold type.

Author	Aneurysm Location	TBO Occlusion Time	Additional Techniques	Complete Occlusion	Complications
Kinjo T. et al. [41] 1986	**Giant BA aneurysm**	N/A	Sendai cocktail Temporary clips on basilar artery and bilateral PCA	N/A	**None**
Shucart W.A. et al. [71] 1990	**BA aneurysm** 3 × large paraclinoid ICA aneurysms	3–18 min (mean 12.5 min.)	None	3 × optimal clip placement 1 × clip repositioning	**Transient oculomotor palsy** Oculomotor and abducens palsy Hemiparesis due to vasospasm Aphasia due frontal infarct (Moya Moya disease)
Tamaki N. et al. [76] 1991	Four large and giant carotid-ophthalmic artery aneurysm	N/A	Temporary ICA clipping distal to aneurysm ICA blood aspiration through second catheter	Successful clipping	Transient oculomotor palsy Hemorrhagic infarction Hydrocephalus (n = 2)
Scott J.A. et al. [68] 1991	Large ophthalmic artery aneurysm	1.5 min. per balloon inflation	Temporary ICA clipping distal to aneurysm Suction through distal lumen of occlusion balloon catheter	Successful obliteration	None
Bailes J.E. et al. [4] 1992	**4 BA aneurysms**	N/A	None	Complete obliteration	Intraoperative aneurysm rupture **Transient oculomotor nerve palsy in 3 patients**
Albert F.K. et al. [2] 1993	2 proximal paraclinoid aneurysm	N/A	Suction-decompression Temporary clip distal ICA	N/A	None
Mizoi K. et al. [51] 1993	9 paraclinoid ICA aneurysms	13–50 min. (mean 26.2 min.)	Retrograde suction-decompression Repeated TBO	3 × Clip repositioning (due to narrowing of parent artery) Successful obliteration in all cases	Intraoperative TBO balloon rupture → surgery continued with new balloon →Embolus developed in M1 Segment → Embolectomy through M1 incisio, MCA occlusion for 20 min → aneurysm clipping followed → patient with transient hemiparesis for 6 h

Table 3. Cont.

Author	Aneurysm Location	TBO Occlusion Time	Additional Techniques	Complete Occlusion	Complications
Mizoi K. et al. [52] 1994	5 BA aneurysms (including 1 large & 1 giant)	15–30 min. (mean 22 min.)	None	3 cases successful obliteration 2 × clip repositioning: Finally one case with remnant at the neck, one complete occlusion	Transient abducens nerve palsy Transient hemiparesis
Fahlbusch R. et al. [19] 1997	3 giant paraclinoid ICA aneurysms	2–6 min.	Retrograde suction-decompression	Clip repositioning in all 3 cases (stenosis of parent vessel or incomplete occlusion)	Vasospasm and temporoparietal infarction (hemiparesis and transient dysphasia, deterioration of vision) 1 thromboembolic complication: sensimotor dysphasia, infarct in temporo-parietal region
Hacein-Bey L. et al. [28] 1998	1 large & 1 giant ICA ophthalmic aneurysm	N/A	None	Complete obliteration	None
Arnautovic K.I. et al. [3] 1998	8 giant and 8 large paraclinoid aneurysms	mean 10.7 min.	Distal temporary clip Suction-decompression	In 1 patient clipping was not possible due to calcification of aneurysm neck and wall, no aneurysm collapse achieved → Coiling Successful clipping in 15 cases	Transient oculomotor nerve palsy 2 temporal lobe infarction with new neurological deficit Hydrocephalus and subdural hygroma Ipsilateral ICA intimal dissection and occlusion at balloon side Transient dysphasia (thromboembolic) Cerebral abscess Transient cerebral edema One death due to intraventricular hemorrhage
Ng P-Y. et al. [60] 2000	24 paraclinoid ICA segment aneurysms (13 large & 11 giant)	2–27 min. (mean 13 min.)	Suction-decompression in 16 cases	Clip adjustment in 7 cases (residual filling of aneurysm and 4 ICA compromise) Complete obliteration in 20 cases, greater than 90% occlusion in 22 cases	1 major MCA infarct related to catheter thromboembolism vasospasm in 3 cases with delayed ischemia 2 deaths (one from fatal MCA infarct)
Thorell W. et al. [80] 2004	6 paraclinoid giant or complex ICA aneurysms	Balloon inflation time less than 3 min. in all cases	None	In 4 patients, navigation of the balloon into intracranial circulation due to carotid tortuosity was not possible All aneurysms were complete occluded	Lumbar drain due to subgaleal CSF collection Lacunar infarction ipsilateral 6 weeks after surgery with mild transient hemiparesis
Steiger H.J. et al. [74] 2005	2 giant carotid opthalmic aneurysms	16 + 24 min. (mean 20 min.)	None	Case 1: Complete occlusion of the intracranial aneurysm part at surgery and 5 months later, endovascular occlusion of infraclinoid aspect of aneurysm Case 2: Small remnant at the neck for patency of parent vessel	Acceleration of vasospasms 15 h after surgery and transient hemiparesis in one case, resolved with hypertensive therapy

Table 3. Cont.

Author	Aneurysm Location	TBO Occlusion Time	Additional Techniques	Complete Occlusion	Complications
Ricci G. et al. [65] 2005	5 giant paraclinoidal ICA aneurysms **1 giant vertebrobasilar junction aneurysm**	N/A	None	Aneurysm obliteration achieved in all cases	None
Parkinson R.J. et al. [63] 2006	Giant paraclinoid ICA aneurysm	N/A	Suction-decompression Temporary clip distal to aneurysm	Complete occlusion and reconstruction of parent vessel	None
Petralia B. et al. [64] 2006	10 giant paraclinoid ICA aneurysm **3 giant vertebrobasilar aneurysm**	15–20 min.	None	All aneurysm excluded with parent vessel patency One balloon rupture One patient underwent coiling at recurrence	None
Hoh D.J. et al. [32] 2008	Large paraclinoid aneurysm	11 min.	Retrograde suction-decompression Temporary clip distal to aneurysm	Aneurysm completely occluded	None
Fulkerson D.H. et al. [23] 2008	63 opthalmic artery aneurysm (26 small, 23 large, 14 giant)	N/A	Temporary clip distal to aneurysm Suction-decompression	N/A	Stroke Hematoma requiring treatment Intraoperative aneurysm rupture New visual deficit 5 deaths
Elhammady M.S. et al. [16] 2009	Large paraclinoid aneurysm	20 min.	Prior attempt for with temporary clipping, thereafter aneurysm rupture and switch to TBO as salvage technique	Complete obliteration	Hemiparesis due to stroke in the inferior division of MCA Vasospasm requiring intra-arterial nicardipine infusion
Skrap M. et al. [72] 2010	11 giant paraclinoid aneurysm **4 vertebrobasilar aneurysm**	15–20 min. (Average 17 min.) Max 5 min. per balloon inflation	One balloon below the aneurysm neck and another in the PCA to stop retrograde flow from ICA	One balloon rupture intraop One clip repositioning in BA Complete occlusion in all cases	None
Dehdashti A.R [13] 2015	Large ophthalmic artery aneurysm	N/A	Temporary clip distal to aneurysm (Pcomm and ICA)	Complete occlusion and patent ophthalmic artery	None

Table 3. *Cont.*

Author	Aneurysm Location	TBO Occlusion Time	Additional Techniques	Complete Occlusion	Complications
Matano F. et al. [49] 2017	2 large ICPC aneurysms	N/A	STA-MCA Bypass prior to clipping Temporary clips on M1, A1 and Pcomm Retrograde suction decompression	Complete occlusion of aneurysms and patent parent vessel	None
Capo G. et al. [11] 2018	**Giant VA aneurysm**	N/A	Temporary clip on PICA	Complete aneurysm occlusion	Transient dysphonia Transient dysphagia Facial nerve palsy PICA occlusion
Xu F. et al. [69] 2018	Large paraclinoid aneurysm	N/A	Temporary clip on Pcomm Retrograde suction-decompression	Complete obliteration of aneurysm	None

TBO = temporary balloon occlusion, PCA = posterior cerebral artery, N/A = not available, BA = basilar artery, min = minutes, TBO = temporary balloon occlusion, ICA = internal carotid artery, MCA = middle cerebral artery, CSF = cerebro-spinal fluid, ICPC = internal carotid posterior communicating artery aneurysms, Pcomm = posterior communicating artery aneurysm, VA = vertebral artery, PICA = posterior inferior cerebellar artery.

Thromboembolic events may be reduced by limiting TBO duration and using double-lumen balloon systems that allow for maintaining continuous heparinized saline catheter flush. In thrombosed aneurysms or patients with severe atherosclerosis, the risk for thromboembolism might be increased. No complications occurred in our series that had a mean TBO time of 10 min. Several series suggested multiple short inflation times of 1.5–5 min to reduce thromboembolic event rate [63,65,78]. Some studies used a preoperative TBO test [83] to investigate the capacity of collateral support. In view of the short TBO time in our series, it is questionable if this is needed. The advantage of performing a TBO procedure in the hybrid OR is that control angiography is possible immediately after clip placement. We performed 2D and 3D intraoperative angiography in the hybrid OR and confirmed aneurysm occlusion in all cases. This standardized protocol can achieve better outcomes [84,85].

The main limitation of our study is the small sample size, as we chose to report on posterior circulation aneurysms only.

5. Conclusions

Intraoperative endovascular TBO is a feasible, safe, and valuable procedure for surgical treatment of complex posterior circulation aneurysm undergoing clipping. In addition, intraoperative DSA and 3D-DSA in the hOR was confirmed as a valuable tool for the evaluation of aneurysm occlusion and possible aneurysm remnants.

Author Contributions: J.F., J.C.K., J.F., L.R. methodology; Software, L.R., M.D.; Validation, J.F., L.R., J.C.K., Y.Y. and M.D.; Formal analysis, J.F.; Writing—original draft preparation, J.C.K., J.F.; Writing—review and editing, J.F., S.M.; Supervision, J.F., L.R. All authors have read and agreed to the published version of the manuscript.

Funding: This research received no external funding.

Conflicts of Interest: The authors declare no conflict of interest.

References

1. Batjer, H.H.; Samson, D.S. Retrograde suction decompression of giant paraclinoidal aneurysms. Technical note. *J. Neurosurg.* **1990**, *73*, 305–306. [CrossRef] [PubMed]
2. Batjer, H.H.; Kopitnik, T.A.; Giller, C.A.; Samson, D.S. Surgery for paraclinoidal carotid artery aneurysms. *J. Neurosurg.* **1994**, *80*, 650–658. [CrossRef] [PubMed]
3. Vlak, M.H.; Rinkel, G.J.; Greebe, P.; van der Bom, J.G.; Algra, A. Trigger factors for rupture of intracranial aneurysms in relation to patient and aneurysm characteristics. *J. Neurol.* **2012**, *259*, 1298–1302. [CrossRef]
4. Brisman, J.L.; Song, J.K.; Newell, D.W. Cerebral aneurysms. *N. Engl. J. Med.* **2006**, *355*, 928–939. [CrossRef] [PubMed]
5. Molyneux, A.J.; Kerr, R.S.; Yu, L.M.; Clarke, M.; Sneade, M.; Yarnold, J.A.; Sandercock, P.; International Subarachnoid Aneurysm Trial Collaborative Group. International subarachnoid aneurysm trial (ISAT) of neurosurgical clipping versus endovascular coiling in 2143 patients with ruptured intracranial aneurysms: A randomised comparison of effects on survival, dependency, seizures, rebleeding, subgroups, and aneurysm occlusion. *Lancet* **2005**, *366*, 809–817. [PubMed]
6. Greving, J.P.; Wermer, M.J.; Brown, R.D., Jr.; Morita, A.; Juvela, S.; Yonekura, M.; Ishibashi, T.; Torner, J.C.; Nakayama, T.; Rinkel, G.J.; et al. Development of the PHASES score for prediction of risk of rupture of intracranial aneurysms: A pooled analysis of six prospective cohort studies. *Lancet Neurol.* **2014**, *13*, 59–66. [CrossRef]
7. Etminan, N.; Brown, R.D., Jr.; Beseoglu, K.; Juvela, S.; Raymond, J.; Morita, A.; Torner, J.C.; Derdeyn, C.P.; Raabe, A.; Mocco, J.; et al. The unruptured intracranial aneurysm treatment score: A multidisciplinary consensus. *Neurology* **2015**, *85*, 881–889. [CrossRef]
8. Nanda, A.; Sonig, A.; Banerjee, A.D.; Javalkar, V.K. Microsurgical management of basilar artery apex aneurysms: A single surgeon's experience from Louisiana State University, Shreveport. *World Neurosurg.* **2014**, *82*, 118–129. [CrossRef]
9. Hernesniemi, J.; Goehre, F. Approaches to upper basilar artery aneurysms. *World Neurosurg.* **2014**, *82*, 1001–1002. [CrossRef]

10. Batjer, H.; Samson, D. Intraoperative aneurysmal rupture: Incidence, outcome, and suggestions for surgical management. *Neurosurgery* **1986**, *18*, 701–707. [CrossRef]
11. Molyneux, A.; Kerr, R.; Stratton, I.; Sandercock, P.; Clarke, M.; Shrimpton, J.; Holman, R.; International Subarachnoid Aneurysm Trial Collaborative Group. International Subarachnoid Aneurysm Trial (ISAT) of neurosurgical clipping versus endovascular coiling in 2143 patients with ruptured intracranial aneurysms: A randomised trial. *Lancet* **2002**, *360*, 1267–1274. [CrossRef]
12. Ogilvy, C.S.; Hoh, B.L.; Singer, R.J.; Putman, C.M. Clinical and radiographic outcome in the management of posterior circulation aneurysms by use of direct surgical or endovascular techniques. *Neurosurgery* **2002**, *51*, 14–21; discussion 21–22. [CrossRef] [PubMed]
13. Krisht, A.F.; Bikmaz, K.; Kadri, P.A.; Partington, S. Outcome of Surgical Clipping of 40 Complex Basilar Aneurysms Using the Transcavernous Route: Paper 34. *Neurosurgery* **2006**, *58*, 407. [CrossRef]
14. Eskridge, J.M.; Song, J.K. Endovascular embolization of 150 basilar tip aneurysms with Guglielmi detachable coils: Results of the Food and Drug Administration multicenter clinical trial. *J. Neurosurg.* **1998**, *89*, 81–86. [CrossRef]
15. Bavinzski, G.; Killer, M.; Gruber, A.; Reinprecht, A.; Gross, C.E.; Richling, B. Treatment of basilar artery bifurcation aneurysms by using Guglielmi detachable coils: A 6-year experience. *J. Neurosurg.* **1999**, *90*, 843–852. [CrossRef]
16. Tateshima, S.; Murayama, Y.; Gobin, Y.P.; Duckwiler, G.R.; Guglielmi, G.; Vinuela, F. Endovascular treatment of basilar tip aneurysms using Guglielmi detachable coils: Anatomic and clinical outcomes in 73 patients from a single institution. *Neurosurgery* **2000**, *47*, 1332–1339; discussion 1339–1342. [CrossRef]
17. Henkes, H.; Fischer, S.; Mariushi, W.; Weber, W.; Liebig, T.; Miloslavski, E.; Brew, S.; Kuhne, D. Angiographic and clinical results in 316 coil-treated basilar artery bifurcation aneurysms. *J. Neurosurg.* **2005**, *103*, 990–999. [CrossRef]
18. Owen, C.M.; Montemurro, N.; Lawton, M.T. Microsurgical Management of Residual and Recurrent Aneurysms After Coiling and Clipping: An Experience With 97 Patients. *Neurosurgery* **2015**, *62* (Suppl. 1), 92–102. [CrossRef]
19. Spetzler, R.F.; McDougall, C.G.; Zabramski, J.M.; Albuquerque, F.C.; Hills, N.K.; Russin, J.J.; Partovi, S.; Nakaji, P.; Wallace, R.C. The Barrow Ruptured Aneurysm Trial: 6-year results. *J. Neurosurg.* **2015**, *123*, 609–617. [CrossRef]
20. Ferns, S.P.; Sprengers, M.E.; van Rooij, W.J.; Rinkel, G.J.; van Rijn, J.C.; Bipat, S.; Sluzewski, M.; Majoie, C.B. Coiling of intracranial aneurysms: A systematic review on initial occlusion and reopening and retreatment rates. *Stroke* **2009**, *40*, e523–e529. [CrossRef]
21. van Eijck, M.; Bechan, R.S.; Sluzewski, M.; Peluso, J.P.; Roks, G.; van Rooij, W.J. Clinical and Imaging Follow-Up of Patients with Coiled Basilar Tip Aneurysms Up to 20 Years. *AJNR Am. J. Neuroradiol.* **2015**, *36*, 2108–2113. [CrossRef] [PubMed]
22. Molyneux, A.J.; Kerr, R.S.; Birks, J.; Ramzi, N.; Yarnold, J.; Sneade, M.; Rischmiller, J.; Collaborators, I. Risk of recurrent subarachnoid haemorrhage, death, or dependence and standardised mortality ratios after clipping or coiling of an intracranial aneurysm in the International Subarachnoid Aneurysm Trial (ISAT): Long-term follow-up. *Lancet Neurol.* **2009**, *8*, 427–433. [CrossRef]
23. Ferns, S.P.; Sprengers, M.E.; van Rooij, W.J.; van Zwam, W.H.; de Kort, G.A.; Velthuis, B.K.; Schaafsma, J.D.; van den Berg, R.; Sluzewski, M.; Brouwer, P.A.; et al. Late reopening of adequately coiled intracranial aneurysms: Frequency and risk factors in 400 patients with 440 aneurysms. *Stroke* **2011**, *42*, 1331–1337. [CrossRef] [PubMed]
24. Juvela, S.; Porras, M.; Heiskanen, O. Natural history of unruptured intracranial aneurysms: A long-term follow-up study. *J. Neurosurg.* **1993**, *79*, 174–182. [CrossRef] [PubMed]
25. Juvela, S.; Porras, M.; Poussa, K. Natural history of unruptured intracranial aneurysms: Probability of and risk factors for aneurysm rupture. *J. Neurosurg.* **2000**, *93*, 379–387. [CrossRef]
26. Wiebers, D.O.; Whisnant, J.P.; Huston, J., III; Meissner, I.; Brown, R.D., Jr.; Piepgras, D.G.; Forbes, G.S.; Thielen, K.; Nichols, D.; O'Fallon, W.M.; et al. Unruptured intracranial aneurysms: Natural history, clinical outcome, and risks of surgical and endovascular treatment. *Lancet* **2003**, *362*, 103–110. [CrossRef]

27. Molyneux, A.J.; Birks, J.; Clarke, A.; Sneade, M.; Kerr, R.S. The durability of endovascular coiling versus neurosurgical clipping of ruptured cerebral aneurysms: 18 year follow-up of the UK cohort of the International Subarachnoid Aneurysm Trial (ISAT). *Lancet* **2015**, *385*, 691–697. [CrossRef]
28. Investigators, U.J.; Morita, A.; Kirino, T.; Hashi, K.; Aoki, N.; Fukuhara, S.; Hashimoto, N.; Nakayama, T.; Sakai, M.; Teramoto, A.; et al. The natural course of unruptured cerebral aneurysms in a Japanese cohort. *N. Engl. J. Med.* **2012**, *366*, 2474–2482. [CrossRef]
29. Sekhar, L.N.; Tariq, F.; Morton, R.P.; Ghodke, B.; Hallam, D.K.; Barber, J.; Kim, L.J. Basilar tip aneurysms: A microsurgical and endovascular contemporary series of 100 patients. *Neurosurgery* **2013**, *72*, 284–298; discussion 298–299. [CrossRef]
30. Hernesniemi, J.; Korja, M. At the apex of cerebrovascular surgery–basilar tip aneurysms. *World Neurosurg.* **2014**, *82*, 37–39. [CrossRef]
31. Yasargil, M.G.; Antic, J.; Laciga, R.; Jain, K.K.; Hodosh, R.M.; Smith, R.D. Microsurgical pterional approach to aneurysms of the basilar bifurcation. *Surg. Neurol.* **1976**, *6*, 83–91. [PubMed]
32. Drake, C.G. Bleeding aneurysms of the basilar artery. Direct surgical management in four cases. *J. Neurosurg.* **1961**, *18*, 230–238. [CrossRef] [PubMed]
33. Tjahjadi, M.; Kivelev, J.; Serrone, J.C.; Maekawa, H.; Kerro, O.; Jahromi, B.R.; Lehto, H.; Niemela, M.; Hernesniemi, J.A. Factors Determining Surgical Approaches to Basilar Bifurcation Aneurysms and Its Surgical Outcomes. *Neurosurgery* **2016**, *78*, 181–191. [CrossRef] [PubMed]
34. Day, J.D.; Fukushima, T.; Giannotta, S.L. Cranial base approaches to posterior circulation aneurysms. *J. Neurosurg.* **1997**, *87*, 544–554. [CrossRef]
35. Hsu, F.P.; Clatterbuck, R.E.; Spetzler, R.F. Orbitozygomatic approach to basilar apex aneurysms. *Neurosurgery* **2005**, *56* (Suppl. 1), 172–177. [CrossRef]
36. Gonzalez, L.F.; Amin-Hanjani, S.; Bambakidis, N.C.; Spetzler, R.F. Skull base approaches to the basilar artery. *Neurosurg. Focus* **2005**, *19*, E3. [CrossRef]
37. Kawase, T.; Toya, S.; Shiobara, R.; Mine, T. Transpetrosal approach for aneurysms of the lower basilar artery. *J. Neurosurg.* **1985**, *63*, 857–861. [CrossRef]
38. Kato, Y.; Sano, H.; Behari, S.; Kumar, S.; Nagahisa, S.; Iwata, S.; Kanno, T. Surgical clipping of basilar aneurysms: Relationship between the different approaches and the surgical corridors. *Minim. Invasive Neurosurg. MIN* **2002**, *45*, 142–145. [CrossRef]
39. Spiessberger, A.; Strange, F.; Fandino, J.; Marbacher, S. Microsurgical Clipping of Basilar Apex Aneurysms: A Systematic Historical Review of Approaches and their Results. *World Neurosurg.* **2018**, *114*, 305–316. [CrossRef]
40. Groff, M.W.; Adams, D.C.; Kahn, R.A.; Kumbar, U.M.; Yang, B.Y.; Bederson, J.B. Adenosine-induced transient asystole for management of a basilar artery aneurysm. Case report. *J. Neurosurg.* **1999**, *91*, 687–690. [CrossRef]
41. Lawton, M.T.; Raudzens, P.A.; Zabramski, J.M.; Spetzler, R.F. Hypothermic circulatory arrest in neurovascular surgery: Evolving indications and predictors of patient outcome. *Neurosurgery* **1998**, *43*, 10–20; discussion 20–21. [CrossRef]
42. Samson, D.; Batjer, H.H.; Bowman, G.; Mootz, L.; Krippner, W.J., Jr.; Meyer, Y.J.; Allen, B.C. A clinical study of the parameters and effects of temporary arterial occlusion in the management of intracranial aneurysms. *Neurosurgery* **1994**, *34*, 22–28; discussion 28–29. [PubMed]
43. Elhammady, M.S.; Nakaji, P.; Farhat, H.; Morcos, J.J.; Aziz-Sultan, M.A. Balloon-assisted clipping of a large paraclinoidal aneurysm: A salvage procedure. *Neurosurgery* **2009**, *65*, E1210–E1211; discussion E1211. [CrossRef] [PubMed]
44. Fandino, J.; Taussky, P.; Marbacher, S.; Muroi, C.; Diepers, M.; Fathi, A.R.; Remonda, L. The concept of a hybrid operating room: Applications in cerebrovascular surgery. *Acta Neurochir. Suppl.* **2013**, *115*, 113–117. [PubMed]
45. Sanai, N.; Tarapore, P.; Lee, A.C.; Lawton, M.T. The current role of microsurgery for posterior circulation aneurysms: A selective approach in the endovascular era. *Neurosurgery* **2008**, *62*, 1236–1249; discussion 1249–1253. [CrossRef] [PubMed]
46. Lawton, M.T.; Abla, A.A.; Rutledge, W.C.; Benet, A.; Zador, Z.; Rayz, V.L.; Saloner, D.; Halbach, V.V. Bypass Surgery for the Treatment of Dolichoectatic Basilar Trunk Aneurysms: A Work in Progress. *Neurosurgery* **2016**, *79*, 83–99. [CrossRef]

47. Basma, J.; Ryttlefors, M.; Latini, F.; Pravdenkova, S.; Krisht, A. Mobilization of the transcavernous oculomotor nerve during basilar aneurysm surgery: Biomechanical bases for better outcome. *Neurosurgery* **2014**, *10* (Suppl. 1), 106–114; discussion 114–115. [CrossRef]
48. Shi, X.; Qian, H.; Singh, K.C.; Zhang, Y.; Zhou, Z.; Sun, Y.; Liu, F. Surgical management of vertebral and basilar artery aneurysms: A single center experience in 41 patients. *Acta Neurochir. (Wien)* **2013**, *155*, 1087–1093. [CrossRef]
49. Yanagisawa, T.; Kinouchi, H.; Sasajima, T.; Shimizu, H. Long-Term Follow-Up for a Giant Basilar Trunk Aneurysm Surgically Treated by Proximal Occlusion and External Carotid Artery to Posterior Cerebral Artery Bypass Using a Saphenous Vein Graft. *J. Stroke Cerebrovasc. Dis.* **2016**, *25*, e212–e213. [CrossRef]
50. Indo, M.; Oya, S.; Matsui, T. Ruptured Basilar Tip Aneurysm in a Patient with Bilateral Internal Carotid Artery Occlusion Successfully Treated with Bilateral Superficial Temporal Artery-Middle Cerebral Artery Anastomoses: Case Report. *World Neurosurg.* **2016**, *86*, 512.e5–512.e8. [CrossRef]
51. Kai, Y.; Hamada, J.; Morioka, M.; Yano, S.; Hamasaki, K.; Ushio, Y. Successful treatment of a ruptured dissecting basilar artery aneurysm. Case report. *J. Neurosurg.* **2004**, *100*, 1072–1075. [CrossRef] [PubMed]
52. Krisht, A.F.; Krayenbuhl, N.; Sercl, D.; Bikmaz, K.; Kadri, P.A. Results of microsurgical clipping of 50 high complexity basilar apex aneurysms. *Neurosurgery* **2007**, *60*, 242–250; discussion 250–252. [CrossRef] [PubMed]
53. Tanaka, Y.; Kobayashi, S.; Hongo, K.; Tada, T.; Nagashima, H.; Kakizawa, Y. Intentional body clipping of wide-necked basilar artery bifurcation aneurysms. *J. Neurosurg.* **2000**, *93*, 169–174. [CrossRef] [PubMed]
54. Matsukawa, H.; Tanikawa, R.; Kamiyama, H.; Tsuboi, T.; Noda, K.; Ota, N.; Miyata, S.; Tokuda, S. Localization in the Interpeduncular Cistern as Risk Factors for the Thalamoperforators' Ischemia, Poor Outcome, and Oculomotor Nerve Palsy in Patients with Complex Unruptured Basilar Apex Aneurysm Treated with Neck Clipping. *World Neurosurg.* **2015**, *84*, 475–482. [CrossRef] [PubMed]
55. Mooney, M.A.; Kalani, M.Y.; Nakaji, P.; Albuquerque, F.C.; McDougall, C.G.; Spetzler, R.F.; Zabramski, J.M. Long-term Patient Outcomes After Microsurgical Treatment of Blister-Like Aneurysms of the Basilar Artery. *Neurosurgery* **2015**, *11* (Suppl. 3), 387–393. [CrossRef]
56. Griessenauer, C.J.; Poston, T.L.; Shoja, M.M.; Mortazavi, M.M.; Falola, M.; Tubbs, R.S.; Fisher, W.S., III. The impact of temporary artery occlusion during intracranial aneurysm surgery on long-term clinical outcome: Part I. Patients with subarachnoid hemorrhage. *World Neurosurg.* **2014**, *82*, 140–148. [CrossRef]
57. Taylor, C.L.; Selman, W.R.; Kiefer, S.P.; Ratcheson, R.A. Temporary vessel occlusion during intracranial aneurysm repair. *Neurosurgery* **1996**, *39*, 893–905; discussion 905–906.
58. Steinberg, G.K.; Drake, C.G.; Peerless, S.J. Deliberate basilar or vertebral artery occlusion in the treatment of intracranial aneurysms. Immediate results and long-term outcome in 201 patients. *J. Neurosurg.* **1993**, *79*, 161–173. [CrossRef]
59. Al-Mousa, A.; Bose, G.; Hunt, K.; Toma, A.K. Adenosine-assisted neurovascular surgery: Initial case series and review of literature. *Neurosurg. Rev.* **2019**, *42*, 15–22. [CrossRef]
60. Desai, V.R.; Rosas, A.L.; Britz, G.W. Adenosine to facilitate the clipping of cerebral aneurysms: Literature review. *Stroke Vasc. Neurol.* **2017**, *2*, 204–209. [CrossRef]
61. Mack, W.J.; Ducruet, A.F.; Angevine, P.D.; Komotar, R.J.; Shrebnick, D.B.; Edwards, N.M.; Smith, C.R.; Heyer, E.J.; Monyero, L.; Connolly, E.S., Jr.; et al. Deep hypothermic circulatory arrest for complex cerebral aneurysms: Lessons learned. *Neurosurgery* **2007**, *60*, 815–827. [CrossRef] [PubMed]
62. Konczalla, J.; Platz, J.; Fichtlscherer, S.; Mutlak, H.; Strouhal, U.; Seifert, V. Rapid ventricular pacing for clip reconstruction of complex unruptured intracranial aneurysms: Results of an interdisciplinary prospective trial. *J. Neurosurg.* **2018**, *128*, 1741–1752. [CrossRef] [PubMed]
63. Skrap, M.; Petralia, B.; Toniato, G. Temporary balloon occlusion during the surgical treatment of giant paraclinoid and vertebrobasilar aneurysms. *Acta Neurochir. (Wien)* **2010**, *152*, 435–442. [CrossRef] [PubMed]
64. Mizoi, K.; Yoshimoto, T.; Takahashi, A.; Ogawa, A. Direct clipping of basilar trunk aneurysms using temporary balloon occlusion. *J. Neurosurg.* **1994**, *80*, 230–236. [CrossRef] [PubMed]
65. Thorell, W.; Rasmussen, P.; Perl, J.; Masaryk, T.; Mayberg, M. Balloon-assisted microvascular clipping of paraclinoid aneurysms. Technical note. *J. Neurosurg.* **2004**, *100*, 713–716. [CrossRef]

66. MacDonald, J.D.; Gyorke, A.; Jacobs, J.M.; Mohammad, S.F.; Sunderland, P.M.; Reichman, M.V. Acute phase vascular endothelial injury: A comparison of temporary arterial occlusion using an endovascular occlusive balloon catheter versus a temporary aneurysm clip in a pig model. *Neurosurgery* **1994**, *34*, 876–881; discussion 881. [CrossRef]
67. Kinjo, T.; Mizoi, K.; Takahashi, A.; Yoshimoto, T.; Suzuki, J. A successfully treated case of giant basilar artery aneurysm utilizing balloon catheter occlusion and brain protective substances. *No Shinkei Geka* **1986**, *14* (Suppl. 3), 397–402.
68. Shucart, W.A.; Kwan, E.S.; Heilman, C.B. Temporary balloon occlusion of a proximal vessel as an aid to clipping aneurysms of the basilar and paraclinoid internal carotid arteries: Technical note. *Neurosurgery* **1990**, *27*, 116–119. [CrossRef]
69. Xu, F.; Huang, L.; Xu, B.; Gu, Y.; Leng, B. Endovascular Retrograde Suction Decompression-Assisted Clipping of Large Paraclinoid Aneurysm in Hybrid Operating Room: 2-Dimensional Operative Video. *World Neurosurg.* **2018**, *114*, 178. [CrossRef]
70. Ricci, G.; Ricci, A.; Gallucci, M.; Zotta, D.; Scogna, A.; Costagliola, C.; Galzio, R.J. Combined endovascular and microsurgical approach in the treatment of giant paraclinoid and vertebrobasilar aneurysms. *J. Neurosurg. Sci.* **2005**, *49*, 1–6.
71. Ng, P.Y.; Huddle, D.; Gunel, M.; Awad, I.A. Intraoperative endovascular treatment as an adjunct to microsurgical clipping of paraclinoid aneurysms. *J. Neurosurg.* **2000**, *93*, 554–560. [CrossRef] [PubMed]
72. Albert, F.K.; Forsting, M.; Aschoff, A.; Krieger, D.; Kunze, S. Clipping of proximal paraclinoid aneurysms with support of the balloon-catheter "trapping-evacuation" technique. Technical note. *Acta Neurochir. (Wien)* **1993**, *125*, 138–141. [CrossRef] [PubMed]
73. Fulkerson, D.H.; Horner, T.G.; Payner, T.D.; Leipzig, T.J.; Scott, J.A.; Denardo, A.J.; Redelman, K.; Goodman, J.M. Endovascular retrograde suction decompression as an adjunct to surgical treatment of ophthalmic aneurysms: Analysis of risks and clinical outcomes. *Neurosurgery* **2009**, *64* (Suppl. 3), ons107–ons111; discussion ons111–ons112. [CrossRef] [PubMed]
74. Bailes, J.E.; Deeb, Z.L.; Wilson, J.A.; Jungreis, C.A.; Horton, J.A. Intraoperative angiography and temporary balloon occlusion of the basilar artery as an adjunct to surgical clipping: Technical note. *Neurosurgery* **1992**, *30*, 949–953.
75. Petralia, B.; Skrap, M. Temporary Balloon Occlusion during Giant Aneurysm Surgery. A Technical Description. *Interv. Neuroradiol.* **2006**, *12*, 245–250. [CrossRef]
76. Hacein-Bey, L.; Connolly, E.S., Jr.; Mayer, S.A.; Young, W.L.; Pile-Spellman, J.; Solomon, R.A. Complex intracranial aneurysms: Combined operative and endovascular approaches. *Neurosurgery* **1998**, *43*, 1304–1312; discussion 1312–1313.
77. Steiger, H.J.; Lins, F.; Mayer, T.; Schmid-Elsaesser, R.; Stummer, W.; Turowski, B. Temporary aneurysm orifice balloon occlusion as an alternative to retrograde suction decompression for giant paraclinoid internal carotid artery aneurysms: Technical note. *Neurosurgery* **2005**, *56* (Suppl. 2), E442. [CrossRef]
78. Scott, J.A.; Horner, T.G.; Leipzig, T.J. Retrograde suction decompression of an ophthalmic artery aneurysm using balloon occlusion. Technical note. *J. Neurosurg.* **1991**, *75*, 146–147. [CrossRef]
79. Hoh, D.J.; Larsen, D.W.; Elder, J.B.; Kim, P.E.; Giannotta, S.L.; Liu, C.Y. Novel use of an endovascular embolectomy device for retrograde suction decompression-assisted clip ligation of a large paraclinoid aneurysm: Technical case report. *Neurosurgery* **2008**, *62* (Suppl. 2), ONSE412–ONSE413; discussion ONSE413–ONSE414. [CrossRef] [PubMed]
80. Fahlbusch, R.; Nimsky, C.; Huk, W. Open surgery of giant paraclinoid aneurysms improved by intraoperative angiography and endovascular retrograde suction decompression. *Acta Neurochir. (Wien)* **1997**, *139*, 1026–1032. [CrossRef]
81. Arnautovic, K.I.; Al-Mefty, O.; Angtuaco, E. A combined microsurgical skull-base and endovascular approach to giant and large paraclinoid aneurysms. *Surg. Neurol.* **1998**, *50*, 504–518; discussion 518–520. [CrossRef]
82. Mizoi, K.; Takahashi, A.; Yoshimoto, T.; Fujiwara, S.; Koshu, K. Combined endovascular and neurosurgical approach for paraclinoid internal carotid artery aneurysms. *Neurosurgery* **1993**, *33*, 986–992. [PubMed]
83. Capo, G.; Vescovi, M.C.; Toniato, G.; Petralia, B.; Gavrilovic, V.; Skrap, M. Giant vertebral aneurysm: A case report detailing successful treatment with combined stenting and surgery. *Surg. Neurol. Int.* **2018**, *9*, 6. [CrossRef] [PubMed]

84. Marbacher, S.; Kienzler, J.C.; Mendelowitsch, I.; D'Alonzo, D.; Andereggen, L.; Diepers, M.; Remonda, L.; Fandino, J. Comparison of Intra- and Postoperative 3-Dimensional Digital Subtraction Angiography in Evaluation of the Surgical Result After Intracranial Aneurysm Treatment. *Neurosurgery* **2019**, nyz487. [CrossRef] [PubMed]
85. Marbacher, S.; Mendelowitsch, I.; Gruter, B.E.; Diepers, M.; Remonda, L.; Fandino, J. Comparison of 3D intraoperative digital subtraction angiography and intraoperative indocyanine green video angiography during intracranial aneurysm surgery. *J. Neurosurg.* **2018**, *131*, 64–71. [CrossRef] [PubMed]

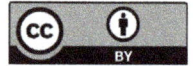

© 2020 by the authors. Licensee MDPI, Basel, Switzerland. This article is an open access article distributed under the terms and conditions of the Creative Commons Attribution (CC BY) license (http://creativecommons.org/licenses/by/4.0/).

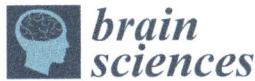

Article

Comparison of Aneurysm Patency and Mural Inflammation in an Arterial Rabbit Sidewall and Bifurcation Aneurysm Model under Consideration of Different Wall Conditions

Basil Erwin Grüter [1,2,*], Stefan Wanderer [1,2], Fabio Strange [1,2], Sivani Sivanrupan [2], Michael von Gunten [3], Hans Rudolf Widmer [4], Daniel Coluccia [1,2], Lukas Andereggen [1,2], Javier Fandino [1,2] and Serge Marbacher [1,2]

1. Department of Neurosurgery, Kantonsspital Aarau, 5000 Aarau, Switzerland; stefan.wanderer@ksa.ch (S.W.); Fabio.Strange@ksa.ch (F.S.); daniel.coluccia@luks.ch (D.C.); lukas.andereggen@ksa.ch (L.A.); javier.fandino@ksa.ch (J.F.); serge.marbacher@ksa.ch (S.M.)
2. Cerebrovascular Research Group, Neurosurgery, Department of BioMedical Research, University of Bern, 3010 Bern, Switzerland; sivani.sivanrupan@students.unibe.ch
3. Institute of Pathology Laenggasse, 3063 Ittigen, Switzerland; mvongunten@patholaenggasse.ch
4. Department of Neurosurgery, Neurocenter and Regenerative Neuroscience Cluster, Inselspital, Bern University Hospital, University of Bern, 3010 Bern, Switzerland; hansrudolf.widmer@insel.ch
* Correspondence: basil.grueter@ksa.ch; Tel.: +41-62-838-41-41

Received: 22 February 2020; Accepted: 25 March 2020; Published: 27 March 2020

Abstract: *Background:* Biological processes that lead to aneurysm formation, growth and rupture are insufficiently understood. Vessel wall inflammation and degeneration are suggested to be the driving factors. In this study, we aimed to investigate the natural course of vital (non-decellularized) and decellularized aneurysms in a rabbit sidewall and bifurcation model. *Methods:* Arterial pouches were sutured end-to-side on the carotid artery of New Zealand White rabbits (vital [$n = 6$] or decellularized [$n = 6$]), and into an end-to-side common carotid artery bifurcation (vital [$n = 6$] and decellularized [$n = 6$]). Patency was confirmed by fluorescence angiography. After 28 days, all animals underwent magnetic resonance and fluorescence angiography followed by aneurysm harvesting for macroscopic and histological evaluation. *Results:* None of the aneurysms ruptured during follow-up. All sidewall aneurysms thrombosed with histological inferior thrombus organization observed in decellularized compared to vital aneurysms. In the bifurcation model, half of all decellularized aneurysms thrombosed whereas the non-decellularized aneurysms remained patent with relevant increase in size compared to baseline. *Conclusions:* Poor thrombus organization in decellularized sidewall aneurysms confirmed the important role of mural cells in aneurysm healing after thrombus formation. Several factors such as restriction by neck tissue, small dimensions and hemodynamics may have prevented aneurysm growth despite pronounced inflammation in decellularized aneurysms. In the bifurcation model, rarefication of mural cells did not increase the risk of aneurysm growth but tendency to spontaneous thrombosis.

Keywords: aneurysm; decellularization; inflammation; rabbits; vessel wall

1. Introduction

In intracerebral aneurysms, the risk of growth and rupture is associated with larger aneurysm size, larger aneurysm height to neck aspect ratio and irregular configuration of the aneurysm [1–3]. However, the biological mechanisms of these morphological characteristics are poorly understood. There is a growing body of evidence that chronic vessel wall inflammation and loss of aneurysm mural cells is a crucial factor in the pathogenesis of aneurysm growth and rupture [4–6]. Aneurysms with vital vessel walls may be able to recruit smooth muscle cells that are able to organize thrombus, to build a neointima and, by phenotype switch, to synthesize extracellular matrix. On the other hand, those aneurysms with a rarefication of cells in their vessel wall seem to be unable to promote aneurysm healing after intraluminal thrombosis. Instead, intra-aneurysmal thrombus may promote chronic inflammation, further weakening of the vessel wall and finally leading to aneurysm growth and rupture [6,7]. This difference becomes fundamentally crucial with endovascular aneurysm treatments, which are conceptually based on a biological healing process, rather than just mechanical flow obstruction [7–9].

The abovementioned putative pathophysiological mechanism was first observed in human samples [10] and later confirmed in an experimental setting in rat saccular sidewall aneurysms [11]. Rabbits stand higher up in the translational chain than rats and allow for experimental creation of complex, more physiological bifurcation aneurysms by means of rheology and hemodynamics [12,13]. Rabbit models are considered ideal for testing of novel endovascular devices, because the rabbit carotid artery is accessible with endovascular devices of the same size as in humans. Therefore, this study aims to investigate the natural course of vital and decellularized aneurysms in a rabbit sidewall and bifurcation aneurysm model with an emphasis on aneurysm patency, growth and mural inflammation.

2. Materials and Methods

New Zealand white rabbits aged 4 months (weighing 3750 ± 293 g) received care in accordance with institutional guidelines. The Committee for Animal Care of the Canton Bern, Switzerland (BE 108/16) approved the experiments. An a priori power analysis was performed, revealing $n = 6$ animals per group needed to reach statistical significance with an estimation of 30% difference between groups. Two animals served as pilots. All animals were randomly allocated to either vital or decellularized aneurysm group. For each group, 6 aneurysms were created. For sidewall aneurysm creation, two animals were used as tissue donors. Two aneurysms (one on each common carotid artery) were created in one animal. For bifurcation aneurysms, only one aneurysm was created per animal. Graft interpositions were taken from the same animal, with no need for additional donor animals.

2.1. Creation of Sidewall Aneurysms

Female rabbits were premedicated with an intramuscular injection of Ketamine HCL 30 mg/kg (Ketalar, 50 mg/mL, Pfizer AG, Zürich Switzerland) and Xylazine 6 mg/kg (Xylapan 20 mg/mL). An auricular vein was then catheterized and a continuous infusion of anesthesia solution (10mL Ketalar and 1.6 mL Xylapan in 50 mL NaCl) was installed with a flow rate of 4–14 mL/h. Furthermore, Fentanyl 1 mg/kg (Fentanyl, Janssen-Cilag, Zug, Switzerland) was applied for analgesia. Animals breathed spontaneously through an oxygen mask. During the operation, animals were located on a heating panel and physiological variables such as heart rate, blood pressure and temperature were continuously monitored. After local infiltration of the pectoral musculature with lidocaine (Lidocaine 1%, Streuli & Co, Uznach, Switzerland), the common carotid artery was dissected on both sides and a previously prepared donor graft (either vital or decellularized) was sutured in an end-to-side configuration, to form a sidewall aneurysm. Nimodipine (Nimotop 0.2 mg/mL, Bayer, Leverkusen, Germany) was locally applied to prevent for vasospasms. A fluorescence angiography was then performed [14,15], to ascertain aneurysm perfusion and patency of the underlying vessel. Afterwards, incised tissues (musculature, subcutaneous and skin) were readapted and closed. Postoperative analgesia was ascertained with transdermal fentanyl application (12 µg/72 h). All animals received postoperative antibiotics by intramuscular injection of terramycin (60 mg/kg), vitamin B12 (Novartis, Basel, Switzerland) 100 mcg subcutaneous and prophylactic low-molecular weight heparin (250 units/kg) subcutaneous.

2.2. Creation of Bifurcation Aneurysm

Due to an internal periodic veterinarian re-evaluation of the standards, anesthesia protocols were slightly adopted for bifurcation models. Premedication comprised subcutaneous application of Ketamine 20 mg/kg, Dexmedetomidine (Novartis, Basel, Switzerland) 100 mg/kg and Methadone (Novartis, Basel, Switzerland) 0.3 mg/kg. Animals were then preoxygenated through a facial mask, before installation of peripheral catheters in the auricular vein and in the contralateral auricular artery. Then, propofol (1–5 mg/kg) (Novartis, Basel, Switzerland) and 0.2–1 mg/kg midazolam (Novartis, Basel, Switzerland) were intravenously administered, followed by intubation with an endotracheal tube (3 mm). Mode of the breathing system was chosen circle, able to be changed from ventilation to spontaneous breathing anytime. A heating pad was continuously used to keep the animals warm during the procedure. For monitoring, a continuous electrocardiogram, a rectal temperature probe and a bispectral index were installed. Analgesia was ascertained by local subcutaneous infiltration with ropivacaine (Novartis, Basel, Switzerland), followed by a continuous rate of infusion of 50 mcg/kg/min lidocaine (Novartis, Basel, Switzerland) and fentanyl boli of 3–10 mcg/kg/h. Postoperatively, Meloxicam 0.5 mg/kg (Novartis, Basel, Switzerland), Vitamin B12 100 mcg (Novartis, Basel, Switzerland) and Clamoxyl 20 mg/kg (Novartis, Basel, Switzerland) were administered subcutaneously. For the first three days, low-molecular weight heparin (250 units/kg) and meloxicam were administered subcutaneously (likewise methadone was administered, if an additive was needed). The detailed surgical technique for creation of bifurcation aneurysms has been presented elsewhere [16]. Briefly, bifurcation aneurysms were created by end-to-side anastomosis of the right common carotid artery to the left common carotid artery and interposition of an arterial pouch, either vital or decellularized.

2.3. A Protocol for Decellularization

Untreated donor arterial grafts with a standardized length of 3–4 mm were taken from a segment of the common carotid artery of a donor animal, ligated with a 6-0 suture on one end and immediately reimplanted in a recipient animal or stored in phosphate buffered saline (PBS) at −4 °C for a maximum of 3 days. All aneurysm pouches were measured, and photo documented on creation and again at follow-up. For decellularization, a modified protocol of a previously described methodology was performed [11,17]: First, grafts were frozen in PBS at −4 °C for several days. Later, they were thawed, rinsed with distilled water and incubated in 1% sodium dodecyl sulphate (SDS) for 6 h at room temperature. The SDS-treated grafts were then washed with gentle shaking and refrozen and kept in PBS at −4 °C until reimplantation. To establish these modifications of the original protocol, various SDS concentration (0.1% and 1%) and several time spans for decellularization (6 h, 9 h,12 h, 15 h and 2 h, 4 h, 6 h, 8 h, respectively) were assessed. All samples were histologically cut and stained with 4′,6-diamidino-2-phenylindole (DAPI) to count nuclei and with hematoxylin-eosin (HE), to assess the integrity of the extracellular matrix such as elastic fibers. Cell nuclei were counted three times for three randomly selected cuts, in each slice specifically for the following wall layers of the vessel: endothelium, media and adventitia. Digital photographs of the microscopic images were taken and analyzed while blinded to the treatment. Near-complete graft decellularization with extracellular fibers still intact was documented after 6 h of 1% SDS treatment.

2.4. Outcome Measurements

After creation, sidewall aneurysms were followed with color coded duplex sonography (SonoSite 180 PLUS, SonoSite, Bothell, WA, USA) on post-operative day 1, day 3 and every 7 days thereof. After a follow-up period of 28 days all animals underwent MRI with MR-angiography (MRA). Immediately afterwards aneurysms were surgically re-exposed, and a fluorescence angiography was performed before euthanasia with an overdose of thiopental (Esconarkon ad us. vet, Streuli & Co, Uznach, Switzerland) and tissue harvesting. Aneurysms were macroscopically inspected and measured. Aneurysm volume was calculated on the basis of a = length, b = width and l = height, with the formula $\pi(1.5(a + b) - \sqrt{ab})(l - b) + (2/3 \times \pi \times ab^2)$. Afterwards fixation in formalin (4% weight/volume solution, J.T. Baker, Arnhem, The Netherlands) and embedding in paraffin for histological analysis followed. Histological staining included HE, Masson–Goldner trichrome, smooth muscle actin, and von Willebrand factor (F8) staining. Stained slices were digitalized (omnyx VL120, GE healthcare,

Chicago, IL, USA) and evaluated with the JVS viewer (JVS view 1.2 full version, University of Tampere, Finland). Histologic scoring was performed blinded to treatment allocation. A 4-scale grading system ("none", "mild", "moderate", "severe") was applied to characterize histology, according to the previously presented neointima score [11].

2.5. Statistics

Data were analyzed and visualized using Graph Pad Prism statistical software 8.3.1 for Windows (GraphPad Software, Sand Diego, CA, USA). Unpaired Mann–Whitney test was used to calculate differences between vital and decellularized aneurysms according to histological analysis with non-parametric values. Values are presented as median with interquartile range and arbitrary units 0–3 representing categories ("none", "mild", "moderate", "severe") according to the neointima score [11]. A *p*-value of <0.05 was considered statistically significant and a *p*-value of <0.001 was considered highly significant.

3. Results

During the study period, no aneurysm ruptured. All sidewall aneurysms (vital and decellularized) thrombosed spontaneously during follow-up. Histologically, inferior thrombus organization was observed in decellularized aneurysms when compared to healing characteristics in vital aneurysms. In the arterial pouch bifurcation model, three out of six aneurysms with decellularized walls thrombosed spontaneously whereas all vital aneurysms (six out of six) stayed patent, with relevant growth pattern in two cases.

3.1. Study and Animal Characteristics

Totally, 22 New Zealand white rabbits were included in this study, weighting 3750 ± 293 g. No animals had to be excluded due to severe comorbidities and no animal died prematurely before planed euthanasia on follow-up day 28. See Figure 1 for an overview of the experimental setting.

For histological evaluation one vital aneurysm in the sidewall constellation and one decellularized aneurysm in the bifurcation constellation was excluded from the final analysis due to insufficient detection of the relevant structures after histologic processing of these heavily scarred aneurysms.

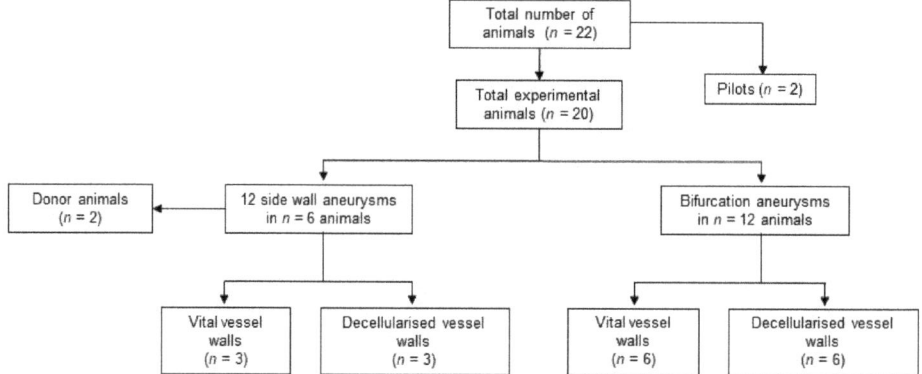

Figure 1. Study design and animal numbers. No animals had to be excluded prematurely for morbidity or mortality.

3.2. Aneurysm Patency

All sidewall aneurysms showed initial flow upon creation but thrombosed within the first two weeks after creation and were not detectable thereafter with either ultrasound or MR angiography. Intraoperative fluorescence angiography confirmed flow obliteration in all these cases. Calculated volume, based on the measured aneurysm size, was significantly smaller for scarred aneurysms at follow-up (7.55 ± 2.73 mm^3) than they were at creation (11.27 ± 3.27 mm^3), $p = 0.0033$ (Figure 2).

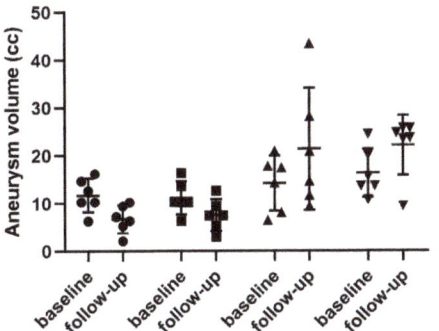

Figure 2. Aneurysm size at baseline and follow-up. Relevant growth pattern was observed in 2 cases of vital bifurcation aneurysms, whereas all the sidewall aneurysms thrombosed spontaneously.

In bifurcation aneurysms, only three out of six aneurysms with decellularized walls thrombosed and all of these with vital vessel walls remained patent until follow-up (exemplary illustration in Figure 3).

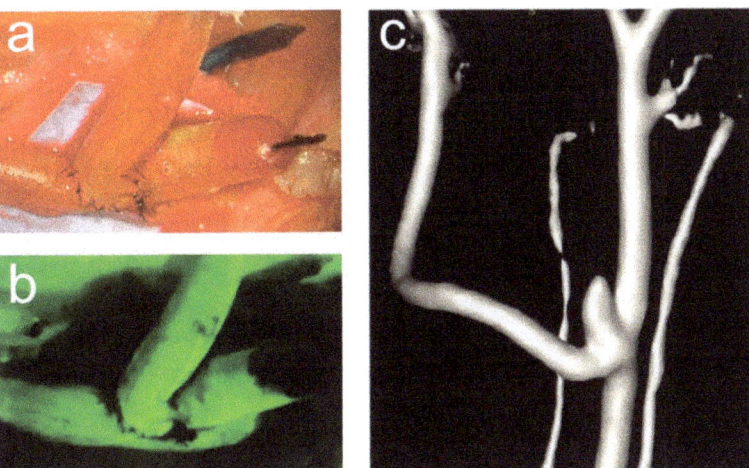

Figure 3. Exemplary illustration of a patent vital bifurcation aneurysm. The operative situs through the operative microscope (a) and the corresponding fluorescence angiography (b) visualize blood flow in both, the aneurysm and the parent artery at the time of aneurysm creation. One-month patency is confirmed by magnetic resonance angiography (c).

Furthermore, these aneurysms showed a pattern of growth from (6.48 ± 1.81 mm^3) on creation to (19.48 mm^3 ± 6.40 mm^3) follow-up ($p = 0.037$)

3.3. Histological Analyses

Overall, there was more inflammation in decellularized aneurysms than in those with vital vessel walls. In sidewall aneurysms, this was reflected by significantly more neutrophil invasion in the thrombus in decellularized than in vital aneurysms ($p = 0.0065$) (Figure 4).

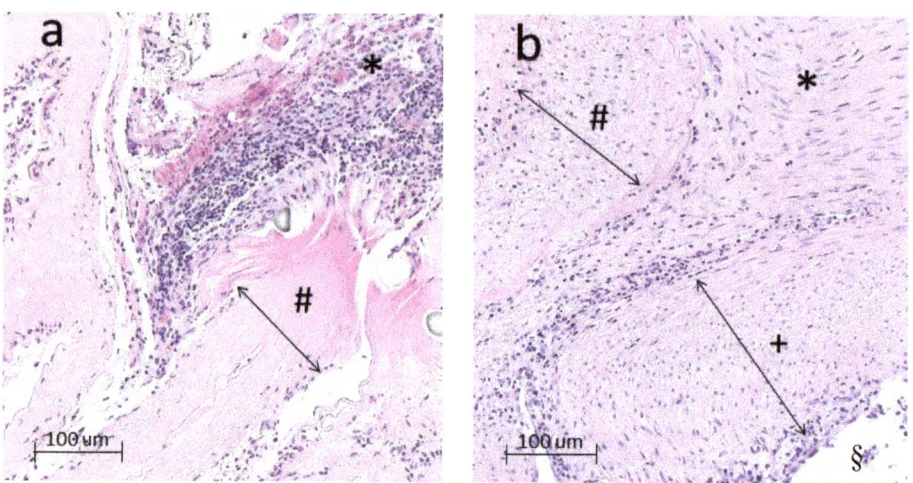

Figure 4. Exemplary histology on a 16-fold digital zoom of a decellularized (**a**) and a vital (**b**) aneurysm in sidewall constellation. The degenerated aneurysm wall (# in a) contains predominantly extracellular matrix fibres only. By contrast, the vital aneurysm wall (# in b) is marked by a high cell density. Inside the thrombus (*) of decellularized aneurysms (**a**), excessive neutrophil infiltration was observed. In (**b**), hardly any neutrophils are visible and derivates of myofibroblast have organized the former intraluminal hematoma into mature thrombus and scare tissue. Furthermore, a thick and consistent neointima (+) separates the former aneurysm cavity from the lumen of the parent artery (§) (similar but no visible in (**a**)).

In bifurcation aneurysm, there were significantly more inflammatory cells (neutrophils) in the wall of decellularized aneurysms compared to vital aneurysms ($p = 0.013$). Periadventitional fibrosis was higher in vital aneurysms than in decellularized ones ($p = 0.013$). All histological characteristics are summarized in Figure 5.

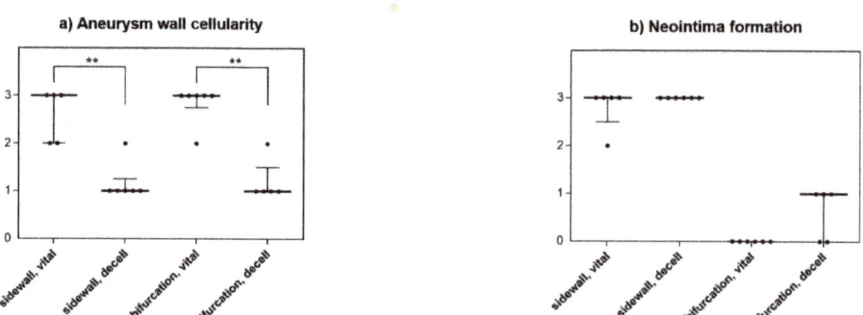

Figure 5. *Cont.*

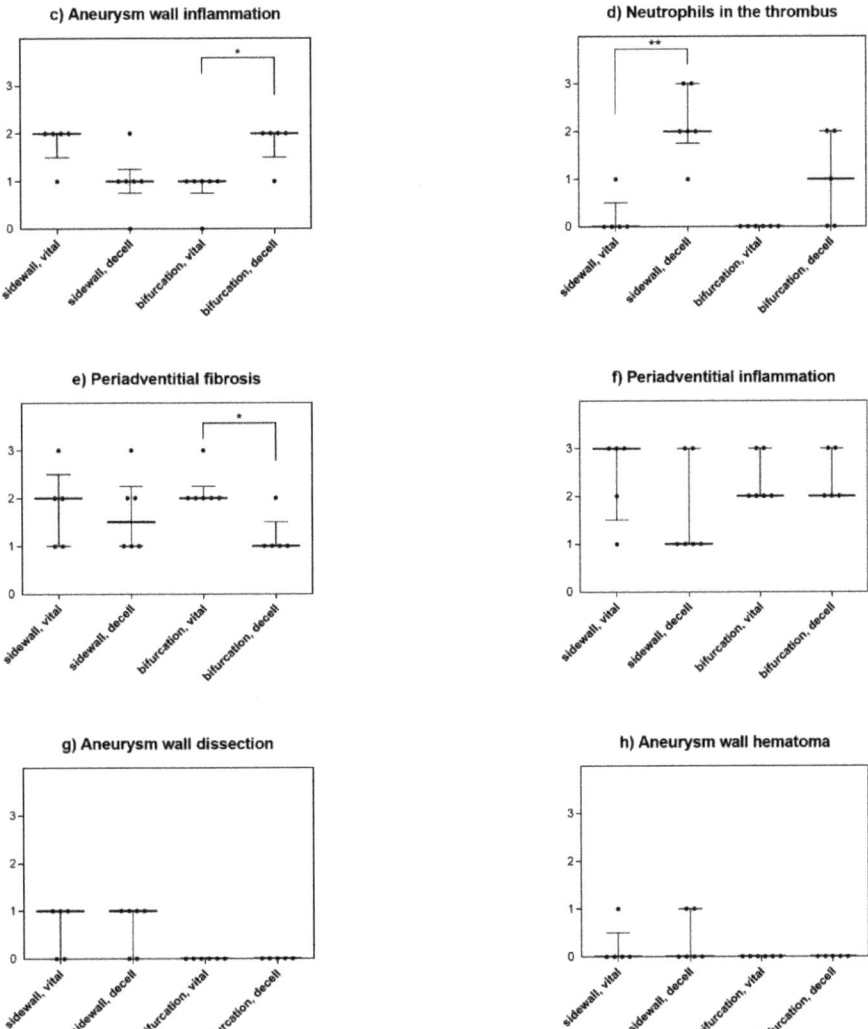

Figure 5. Detailed histological findings for all analyzed features. In both models, aneurysm wall cellularity was significantly lower in decellularized aneurysms than in vital aneurysms, confirming a successful experimental decellularization (**a**). Spontaneous thrombosis and neointima formation (**b**) were strong in the sidewall constellation, but not so in the bifurcation model. In the bifurcation model, aneurysm wall inflammation was significantly more pronounced in decellularized aneurysms when compared with vital aneurysms (**c**). However, there was no difference in terms of aneurysm wall inflammation in the sidewall model. On the other hand, there were significantly more inflammation cells, i.e., neutrophils in the thrombus of decellularized sidewall aneurysms, a difference not as distinctly observed in the bifurcation constellation (**d**). In turn, periadventitial fibrosis was significantly higher in vital than in decellularized bifurcation aneurysms, but not in sidewall aneurysms (**e**). There were no relevant differences for periadventitial inflammation (**f**), aneurysm wall dissection (**g**) or aneurysm wall hematoma (**h**) between different wall conditions for either aneurysm model. A 4-scale grading system 0 = none, 1 = mild, 2 = moderate, 3 = severe was applied to characterize histology [11]. *: $p < 0.05$, ** $p < 0.001$.

4. Discussion

The results of this study demonstrate that all arterial pouch (decellularized and non-decellularized) sidewall aneurysms thrombose spontaneously during follow-up without increase in size. Poor thrombus organization in decellularized sidewall aneurysms confirms the important role of mural cells in aneurysm healing. In the bifurcation aneurysm model, removal of mural cells did not increase the risk of aneurysm growth.

In our experiments, all sidewall aneurysms thrombosed spontaneously without any treatment. This is opposed to the natural course of saccular sidewall aneurysms which were sutured as standardized arterial pouches on the abdominal aorta in a rat model [18]. In that model the authors found a clear pattern of growth in decellularized aneurysms [11]. We hypothesize that the pressure of surrounding muscular tissues in the rabbit neck may counteract the artificially created saccular aneurysms from growth. Furthermore, the base dimensions of these aneurysms are given by the diameter of the carotid artery of the donor animal. This size was usually smaller (approximately 1–1.5 mm) than in a rat aorta (2–3 mm). Together with the different hemodynamics between the rat aorta and the rabbit carotid artery, these aneurysms may have been simply too small for a sufficient perfusion, particularly since the relatively thick and muscular arterial walls may have a tendency to self-contract or increased fibrosis after transplantation. Ding et al. found a patency rate of 95% after 3 weeks in venous pouch sidewall aneurysms on rabbit carotids [19].

In order to overcome these limitation factors, as a next step we repeated the series with non-decellularized and decellularized arterial pouch aneurysms in a hemodynamically more challenging bifurcation constellation. Previous experiments demonstrated in various species (rats, rabbits and dogs) that spontaneous thrombosis occurs less frequently in bifurcation than sidewall venous pouch aneurysms [20–22]. In contrast to these earlier findings, however, all decellularized arterial pouch aneurysms thrombosed even in the setting of an artificial bifurcation. Most previous studies with degenerated vessel walls used elastase eradication of the cells [23–26]. Sodium dodecyl sulfate (SDS) is a detergent that destroys cells but leaves extracellular matrix intact. Its use for experimental decellularization worked well in a previously established rat model, where decellularized aneurysms have been shown to grow over time and eventually rupture, in contrast to aneurysms with vital vessel walls [6,9,11]. However, the completely decellularized graft (including eradication of endothelial cells) after SDS treatment may exhibit prothrombogenic properties. This may be an explanation for the finding of high rate of thrombosed decellularized bifurcation aneurysms. The growing pattern of bifurcation aneurysms with vital vessel walls indicates that the hemodynamic constellation (in a vessel bifurcation) is an important factor for aneurysm enlargement/growth.

When comparing vital and decellularized aneurysms histologically, there was a clear pattern of more pronounced inflammation in decellularized aneurysms for both sidewall and bifurcation aneurysms. This is in line with previous findings [27–29]. For aneurysm healing, intraluminal thrombus needs to undergo gradual organization into a mature thrombus and a neointima needs to form. This process is mediated by smooth muscle cells and myofibroblasts, which migrate into the thrombus, presumably originating in the vessel wall. If there is a substantial diminution in the pool of these cells (i.e., after decellularization) the intraluminal thrombus will undergo cycles of lysis and re-thrombosis instead of scarification [6,11]. This instable thrombus formation causes local inflammatory reactions which promotes further vessel wall weakening.

In summary, there was more pronounced inflammation in decellularized aneurysm than in those with vital walls. However, decellularized aneurysms did not show any pattern of growth or rupture, neither in a sidewall nor in a bifurcation constellation. Therefore, the presented aneurysm models need further refinements to allow for meaningful experiments with a translational focus. Further experiments should use other degrading substances like elastase, test anti-platelet medications to prevent spontaneous thrombus formation, or relocation of the experimental aneurysms into the abdominal cavity to allow for more unrestricted growth. However, with all these issues addressed, still no animal model ever will perfectly match all aspects of the human condition of the disease [30,31].

For instance, there are relevant differences in thrombus formation and endothelial cell coverage between rabbits and humans. In addition, we used healthy arteries in which cells but not the extracellular matrix was destroyed to form aneurysms. However, the elastin content of real aneurysms is inferior to that of healthy arteries [32]. Furthermore, the aneurysm angioarchitecture influences hemodynamic characteristics, and with that the rate of spontaneous thrombosis. Despite all efforts made to standardize aneurysm dimensions and geometry (the latter specifically for either sidewall or bifurcation constellation), we could not avoid differences of few millimeters in size of the vessel pouches and thus in hemodynamics. Further limitations include the relatively small sample size of $n = 6$ animals per group. Lastly, a longer follow-up than 28 days would probably be better to characterize hemodynamic-induced changes in the bifurcation constellation.

5. Conclusions

The results of poor thrombus organization in decellularized rabbit arterial sidewall aneurysms confirm the important role of mural cells in aneurysm healing after intraluminal thrombus formation. Several factors such as restriction by neck tissue, small dimensions and hemodynamics may have prevented aneurysm growth despite pronounced inflammation in decellularized aneurysms. Even in the bifurcation aneurysm model, removal of mural cells did not increase the risk for aneurysm growth but resulted in a higher rate of spontaneous thrombosis. Future studies should examine the role of less thrombogenic degenerated aneurysm wall pouches in a rabbit artificial bifurcation model.

Author Contributions: B.E.G and S.M.: design of the study. B.E.G., F.S., S.W. and S.S. conductance of experiments and collection of data. B.E.G., F.S., S.W. M.v.G. and H.R.W. histological processing and evaluation. D.C., L.A., and J.F. supervision and mentorship. S.M. was in charge of the overall direction. B.E.G. drafted the manuscript with critical inputs from S.W., F.S. and S.M. All authors have read and agreed to the published version of the manuscript.

Funding: This work was supported by research funds of the Research Council, Kantonsspital Aarau, Aarau, Switzerland (FR 1400.000.054). The authors are solely responsible for the design and conduct of the presented study and declare no competing interests.

Acknowledgments: The authors thank Olgica Beslac and Kay Nettelbeck for their technical assistance during the operations and Daniela Casoni DVM, PhD and Alessandra Bergadano, DVM, PhD, for the dedicated veterinary support. Furthermore, we thank Rainer Grobholz for assistance with digitalization of the histology and Monika Werren for her assistance with MR imaging. We are thankful to Adrian Baumgartner for his support with mathematical calculations. Finally, we thank Carline Perren for her help with regulatory and administrative tasks.

Conflicts of Interest: The authors declare no conflict of interest.

References

1. Morita, A.; Kirino, T.; Hashi, K.; Aoki, N.; Fukuhara, S.; Hashimoto, N.; Nakayama, T.; Sakai, M.; Teramoto, A.; Tominari, S.; et al. The natural course of unruptured cerebral aneurysms in a Japanese cohort. *N. Engl. J. Med.* **2012**, *366*, 2474–2482. [PubMed]
2. Wiebers, D.O.; Whisnant, J.P.; Huston, J., III. Unruptured intracranial aneurysms: Natural history, clinical outcome, and risks of surgical and endovascular treatment. *Lancet* **2003**, *362*, 103–110. [CrossRef]
3. Duan, Z.; Li, Y.; Guan, S.; Ma, C.; Han, Y.; Ren, X.; Wei, L.; Li, W.; Lou, J.; Yang, Z. Morphological parameters and anatomical locations associated with rupture status of small intracranial aneurysms. *Sci. Rep.* **2018**, *8*, 6440. [CrossRef] [PubMed]
4. Kataoka, K.; Taneda, M.; Asai, T.; Kinoshita, A.; Ito, M.; Kuroda, R. Structural fragility and inflammatory response of ruptured cerebral aneurysms. A comparative study between ruptured and unruptured cerebral aneurysms. *Stroke J. Cereb. Circ.* **1999**, *30*, 1396–1401. [CrossRef]
5. Frosen, J. Smooth muscle cells and the formation, degeneration, and rupture of saccular intracranial aneurysm wall—A review of current pathophysiological knowledge. *Transl. Stroke Res.* **2014**, *5*, 347–356. [CrossRef] [PubMed]
6. Marbacher, S.; Frosen, J.; Marjamaa, J.; Anisimov, A.; Honkanen, P.; von Gunten, M.; Abo-Ramadan, U.; Hernesniemi, J.; Niemelä, M. Intraluminal cell transplantation prevents growth and rupture in a model of rupture-prone saccular aneurysms. *Stroke J. Cereb. Circ.* **2014**, *45*, 3684–3690. [CrossRef]

7. Marbacher, S.; Niemela, M.; Hernesniemi, J.; Frosen, J. Recurrence of endovascularly and microsurgically treated intracranial aneurysms-review of the putative role of aneurysm wall biology. *Neurosurg. Rev.* **2017**, *42*, 49–58. [CrossRef]
8. Gruter, B.E.; Taschler, D.; Strange, F.; Rey, J.; von Gunten, M.; Grandgirard, D.; Leib, S.L.; Remonda, L.; Widmer, H.R.; Nevzati, E.; et al. Testing bioresorbable stent feasibility in a rat aneurysm model. *J. Neurointerv. Surg.* **2019**. [CrossRef]
9. Nevzati, E.; Rey, J.; Coluccia, D.; Grüter, B.E.; Wanderer, S.; Vongunten, M.; Remonda, L.; Frosen, J.; Widmer, H.R.; Fandino, J.; et al. Aneurysm wall cellularity affects healing after coil embolization: Assessment in a rat saccular aneurysm model. *J. Neurointerv. Surg.* **2019**. [CrossRef]
10. Frosen, J.; Piippo, A.; Paetau, A.; Kangasniemi, M.; Niemelä, M.; Hernesniemi, J.; Jääskeläinen, J. Remodeling of saccular cerebral artery aneurysm wall is associated with rupture: Histological analysis of 24 unruptured and 42 ruptured cases. *Stroke J. Cereb. Circ.* **2004**, *35*, 2287–2293. [CrossRef]
11. Marbacher, S.; Marjamaa, J.; Bradacova, K.; Von Gunten, M.; Honkanen, P.; Abo-Ramadan, U.; Hernesniemi, J.; Niemelä, M.; Frösen, J. Loss of mural cells leads to wall degeneration, aneurysm growth, and eventual rupture in a rat aneurysm model. *Stroke J. Cereb. Circ.* **2014**, *45*, 248–254. [CrossRef] [PubMed]
12. Sherif, C.; Fandino, J.; Erhardt, S.; di Ieva, A.; Killer, M.; Kleinpeter, G.; Marbacher, S. Microsurgical venous pouch arterial-bifurcation aneurysms in the rabbit model: Technical aspects. *JoVE* **2011**. [CrossRef] [PubMed]
13. Marbacher, S.; Erhardt, S.; Schlappi, J.A.; Coluccia, D.; Remonda, L.; Fandino, J.; Sherif, C. Complex bilobular, bisaccular, and broad-neck microsurgical aneurysm formation in the rabbit bifurcation model for the study of upcoming endovascular techniques. *AJNR Am. J. Neuroradiol.* **2011**, *32*, 772–777. [CrossRef] [PubMed]
14. Gruter, B.E.; Taschler, D.; Rey, J.; Strange, F.; Nevzati, E.; Fandino, J.; Marbacher, S.; Coluccia, D. Fluorescence Video Angiography for Evaluation of Dynamic Perfusion Status in an Aneurysm Preclinical Experimental Setting. *Oper. Neurosurg. (Hagerstown)* **2019**, *17*, 432–438. [CrossRef]
15. Strange, F.; Sivanrupan, S.; Gruter, B.E.; Rey, J.; Taeschler, D.; Fandino, J.; Marbacher, S. Fluorescence Angiography for Evaluation of Aneurysm Perfusion and Parent Artery Patency in Rat and Rabbit Aneurysm Models. *JoVE* **2019**. [CrossRef]
16. Wanderer, S.; Grüter, B.E.; Strange, F.; Bertalanffy, H. Microsurgical Creation of Complex Bifurcation Aneurysms with Different Wall Conditions in New Zealand White Rabbits—Introducing the Surgical Technique in a New Animal Model. In Proceedings of the 6th Annual Meeting of the EANS Section of Vascular Neurosurgery, Nice, France, 5–6 September 2019.
17. Allaire, E.; Guettier, C.; Bruneval, P.; Plissonnier, D.; Michel, J.B. Cell-free arterial grafts: Morphologic characteristics of aortic isografts, allografts, and xenografts in rats. *J. Vasc. Surg.* **1994**, *19*, 446–456. [CrossRef]
18. Marbacher, S.; Marjamaa, J.; Abdelhameed, E.; Hernesniemi, J.; Niemela, M.; Frosen, J. The Helsinki rat microsurgical sidewall aneurysm model. *JoVE* **2014**, *92*, e51071. [CrossRef]
19. Ding, Y.H.; Tieu, T.; Kallmes, D.F. Creation of sidewall aneurysm in rabbits: Aneurysm patency and growth follow-up. *J. Neurointerv. Surg.* **2014**, *6*, 29–31. [CrossRef]
20. Nishikawa, M.; Smith, R.D.; Yonekawa, Y. Experimental intracranial aneurysms. *Surg. Neurol.* **1977**, *7*, 241–244.
21. Marbacher, S.; Tastan, I.; Neuschmelting, V.; Erhardt, S.; Coluccia, D.; Sherif, C.; Remonda, L.; Fandino, J. Long-term patency of complex bilobular, bisaccular, and broad-neck aneurysms in the rabbit microsurgical venous pouch bifurcation model. *Neurol. Res.* **2012**, *34*, 538–546. [CrossRef]
22. Kirse, D.J.; Flock, S.; Teo, C.; Rahman, S.; Mrak, R. Construction of a vein-pouch aneurysm at a surgically created carotid bifurcation in the rat. *Microsurgery* **1996**, *17*, 681–689. [CrossRef]
23. Dai, D.; Ding, Y.H.; Kadirvel, R.; Lewis, D.A.; Kallmes, D.F. Experience with microaneurysm formation at the basilar terminus in the rabbit elastase aneurysm model. *AJNR Am. J. Neuroradiol.* **2010**, *31*, 300–303. [CrossRef] [PubMed]
24. Wang, S.; Dai, D.; Kolumam Parameswaran, P.; Kadirvel, R.; Ding, Y.H.; Robertson, A.M.; Kallmes, D.F. Rabbit aneurysm models mimic histologic wall types identified in human intracranial aneurysms. *J. Neurointerv. Surg.* **2018**, *10*, 411–415. [CrossRef] [PubMed]
25. Brinjikji, W.; Ding, Y.H.; Kallmes, D.F.; Kadirvel, R. From bench to bedside: Utility of the rabbit elastase aneurysm model in preclinical studies of intracranial aneurysm treatment. *J. Neurointerv. Surg.* **2016**, *8*, 521–525. [CrossRef]

26. Marbacher, S.; Wanderer, S.; Strange, F.; Grüter, B.E.; Fandino, J. Saccular Aneurysm Models Featuring Growth and Rupture: A Systematic Review. *Brain Sci.* **2020**, *10*, 101. [CrossRef]
27. Chalouhi, N.; Hoh, B.L.; Hasan, D. Review of cerebral aneurysm formation, growth, and rupture. *Stroke J. Cereb. Circ.* **2013**, *44*, 3613–3622. [CrossRef]
28. Krings, T.; Mandell, D.M.; Kiehl, T.R.; Geibprasert, S.; Tymianski, M.; Alvarez, H.; TerBrugge, K.G.; Hans, F.J. Intracranial aneurysms: From vessel wall pathology to therapeutic approach. *Nat. Rev. Neurol.* **2011**, *7*, 547–559. [CrossRef]
29. Chalouhi, N.; Ali, M.S.; Jabbour, P.M.; Tjoumakaris, S.I.; Gonzalez, L.F.; Rosenwasser, R.H.; Koch, W.J.; Dumont, A.S. Biology of intracranial aneurysms: Role of inflammation. *J. Cereb. Blood Flow Metab.* **2012**, *32*, 1659–1676. [CrossRef]
30. Strange, F.; Gruter, B.E.; Fandino, J.; Marbacher, S. Preclinical Intracranial Aneurysm Models: A Systematic Review. *Brain Sci.* **2020**, *10*, 134. [CrossRef]
31. Marbacher, S.; Strange, F.; Frosen, J.; Fandino, J. Preclinical extracranial aneurysm models for the study and treatment of brain aneurysms: A systematic review. *J. Cereb. Blood Flow Metab.* **2020**. Epub ahead of print. [CrossRef]
32. Halabi, C.M.; Kozel, B.A. Vascular elastic fiber heterogeneity in health and disease. *Curr. Opin. Hematol.* **2020**. [CrossRef] [PubMed]

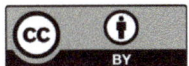

© 2020 by the authors. Licensee MDPI, Basel, Switzerland. This article is an open access article distributed under the terms and conditions of the Creative Commons Attribution (CC BY) license (http://creativecommons.org/licenses/by/4.0/).

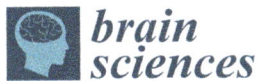

Article

Systemic and CSF Interleukin-1α Expression in a Rabbit Closed Cranium Subarachnoid Hemorrhage Model: An Exploratory Study

Davide Marco Croci [1,2,3,*], Stefan Wanderer [2,4], Fabio Strange [2,4], Basil E. Grüter [2,4], Daniela Casoni [5], Sivani Sivanrupan [2], Hans Rudolf Widmer [6], Stefano Di Santo [6], Javier Fandino [2,4], Luigi Mariani [1] and Serge Marbacher [2,4]

1. Department of Neurosurgery, University Hospital Basel, 4031 Basel, Switzerland; luigi.mariani@usb.ch
2. Cerebrovascular Research Group, Department of BioMedical Research, University of Bern, 3008 Bern, Switzerland; stefan.wanderer@ksa.ch (S.W.); Fabio.strange@ksa.ch (F.S.); bgrueter@gmx.ch (B.E.G.); Sivani.sivanrupan@unibe.ch (S.S.); javier.fandino@ksa.ch (J.F.); Serge.Marbacher@ksa.ch (S.M.)
3. Department of Neurosurgery, Neurocenter of Southern Switzerland, Regional Hospital Lugano, 6900 Lugano, Switzerland
4. Department of Neurosurgery, Kantonsspital Aarau, 5001 Aarau, Switzerland
5. Department of Biomedical Research, University of Bern, 3008 Bern, Switzerland; Daniela.Casoni@unibern.ch
6. Department of Neurosurgery, Bern University Hospital, Inselspital Bern, 3008 Bern, Switzerland; Hansrudolf.widmer@insel.ch (H.R.W.); Stefano.disanto@insel.ch (S.D.S.)
* Correspondence: neurosurgery@ksa.ch or davide.croci@eoc.ch; Tel.: +41-62-838-663; Fax: +41-62-838-66-29

Received: 6 August 2019; Accepted: 23 September 2019; Published: 24 September 2019

Abstract: Background: The inflammatory pathway in cerebrospinal fluid (CSF) leads to delayed cerebral vasospasm (DCVS) and delayed cerebral ischemia (DCI) after subarachnoid hemorrhage (SAH). The role of IL-1α has never been evaluated in a rabbit SAH model. The aim of our study is to analyze systemic and CSF changes of IL-1α, and to evaluate potential associations with the onset of DCVS in a rabbit closed cranium SAH model. Methods: 17 New Zealand white rabbits were randomized into two groups, SAH ($n = 12$) and sham ($n = 5$). In the first group, SAH was induced by extracranial-intracranial shunting from the subclavian artery into the cerebral cistern of magna under intracranial pressure (ICP) monitoring. The sham group served as a control. The CSF and blood samples for IL-1α measurement were taken at day zero before SAH induction and at day three. Results: There was a significant increase of ICP ($p = 0.00009$) and a decrease of cerebral perfusion pressure (CPP) ($p = 0.00089$) during SAH induction. At follow up, there was a significant increase of systemic IL-1α in the SAH as compared with the sham group ($p = 0.042$). There was no statistically significant difference in the CSF values in both groups. The CSF IL-1α values showed a correlation trend of DCVS. Conclusions: Systemic IL-1α levels are elevated after SAH induction in a rabbit SAH model.

Keywords: subarachnoid hemorrhage; IL-1α; inflammation; animal model

1. Introduction

Delayed cerebral vasospasm (DCVS) and delayed cerebral ischemia (DCI) are severe complications of subarachnoid hemorrhage (SAH). The inflammatory pathway due to blood hemolysis in cerebrospinal fluid (CSF) has been recognized to be one of the leading factors causing DCVS and DCI. Different cytokines and interleukins have been described as mediators of the inflammation cascade initiated by blood products in the subarachnoid space, leading to DCVS and DCI [1–4]. Interleukin-1 (IL-1) is a family of cytokines which induces a group of different cytokines and the expression of integrins on leukocytes and endothelial cells mediating the inflammatory response [5–7]. IL-1 is produced in different immune cells such as macrophages, lymphocytes, and microglia [8,9]. Despite IL-1 being typically linked to inflammation, it has also been associated with different functions such as insulin secretion, fever induction, and neuronal phenotype development [10–14]. IL-1 has been described to be a key mediator of neuronal injury after acute brain injury [15,16]. Moreover, it usually upregulates the expression of interleukin-6 (IL-6), which triggers local inflammation and activation of the systemic acute phase response. IL-1 stimulates the release of IL-6 from mast cells [17], which have been described to be present in the aneurysm wall of SAH patients and the muscular layer of cerebral arteries [18,19]. The IL-6 concentrations are elevated in the cerebrospinal fluid (CSF) in animal models of SAH and in patients suffering SAH. Moreover, high concentrations of CSF IL-6 correspond to worse clinical outcomes in patients affected by SAH [1,3].

IL-1α and IL-1β are the most known interleukins subtypes in the IL-1 family and both are proinflammatory and bind at the same receptor, the type I IL-1 receptor (IL-1RI). The initiated signaling cascade results in the expression of inflammatory genes [5,6,20]. IL-1α differs mainly from IL-1β in primary structure. IL-1α, in contrast to IL-1β, appears to have bioactivity while in the form of an intact pro-cytokine precursor on the cell surface and intracellularly [21]. The IL-1 receptor antagonist (IL-1Ra) blocks the signaling at the receptor, inhibiting the inflammatory effects of IL-1α and IL-1β [22,23]. IL-1α has an emerging importance in the initiation and maintenance of inflammation in different human diseases and the initiation of the sterile inflammatory response. In ischemic strokes, IL-1α has been described to be expressed early in areas of focal neuronal injury after ischemic injury. In addition, it is chronically elevated in the brain after an experimental stroke, suggesting that it is present during post-stroke angiogenic periods. Moreover, IL-1α not only precedes the expression of IL-1β and IL-6, but it has also been described to be more potent in stimulating the expression of IL-6 [24–26].

Considering that to date no medical treatment has been shown to properly prevent the onset of DCVS and DCI after SAH, the outcome of patients affected by DCVS and DCI after SAH remains very poor. As previously described, the inflammation reaction initiated in early brain injury phase after SAH is highly involved in the development of DCVS and DCI [1,3,18,27]. IL-1α is one of the key player and the earliest interleukins released during the sterile inflammation cascade [24]. A better understanding of this interleukin in the inflammation cascade after SAH could be essential for the development of future target therapies to prevent DCVS and DCI in patients affected by SAH.

With this study, we aimed to evaluate the levels of systemic and CSF IL-1α in an established extracranial intracranial closed rabbit SAH model and to analyze if there are any correlations with DCVS.

2. Materials and Methods

2.1. Animals, Study Design, and Anesthesia

As a subproject of an ongoing study, a total of 17 female New Zealand white rabbits (3.1–4.1 kg body weight, 16 weeks old, Charles River, Sulzfeld, Germany) were previously randomly allocated into two different groups using a web-based randomization system [28], i.e., the SAH group ($n = 12$) and in the sham group ($n = 5$). After the clinical examination, general anesthesia was induced in all rabbits with a mixture of subcutaneous ketamine (Narketan 100 mg/mL, Vetoquinol AG, Bern, Switzerland) (30 mg/kg) and xylazine (6 mg/kg, Xylapan, 20 mg/mL, Vetoquinol AG, Bern, Switzerland). After 15 min under administration of 2–4 L of O_2 through a facial mask, two 22 G intravenous cannulae were inserted in the marginal auricular vein and into the auricular artery, respectively. Perincisional ropivacaine 1% (Sintetica S.A., Mendrisio, Switzerland) was infiltrated into the axillary region (access for the subclavian artery). A supraglottic device was introduced and general anesthesia maintained with isoflurane in oxygen targeting an EtIso of 1.3%. Spontaneous ventilation was allowed. Ringer lactate (4–10 mL/kg/h) was infused through the vein access. Continuous monitoring of heart rate, respiratory rate, oxygen arterial saturation, capnography, invasive blood pressure, non-invasive blood pressure (Doppler technique), esophageal temperature, as well as inspired and expired fraction of gases (air, CO_2 and isoflurane) was provided. During the procedure, at least 1 blood gas was analyzed.

Additional boluses of fentanyl (Fentanyl Syntetica 0.5 mg/10 mL, Sintetica S.A., Mendrisio, Switzerland) were provided (3–10 mcg/kg IV) if nociception was deemed insufficient. Nociception was continuously assessed through cardiovascular monitoring and at intervals of 5 min through stimulation of pedal reflex (toe pinch). Hypothermia was prevented using a warming mattress and hypotension (MAP less than 60 mmHg) was addressed with the use of noradrenaline titrated to effect. Postoperative analgesia was provided with a fentanyl patch (12 mcg/h; Durogesic Matrix 12 µg/h, Janssen-Cilag AG, Schaffausen, Switzerland) put on the outer ears. The animals were carefully observed during the recovery phase. Oxygen supplementation and fluid therapy were provided until sternal recumbency was achieved. Neurological status was assessed at 6, 12, 24, 48, and 72 h post SAH, according to a four-point grading system, as previously described [29].

2.2. Digital Subtraction Angiography and SAH Induction

Detailed protocols for surgery and angiography have been previously described elsewhere [30–32]. Digital subtraction angiography (DSA) was performed under general anesthesia at day 0 prior to SAH and on day 3. The rabbits' subclavian artery was prepared and cannulated with a 5.5 French catheter (Silicone Catheter STH-C040, Connectors Verbindungstechink AG, Tagelswangen, Switzerland). The catheter tip was advanced to the origin of the vertebral artery. Intraarterial bolus injection of contrast dye followed (0.6 mL/kg Iopamidol, Iopamiro, Bracoo Suisse, Mendrisio, Switzerland). Images of the basilar artery were obtained using a rapid sequential angiographic technique (DFP 2000A, Toshiba, Tokyo, Japan). The same procedure was performed at day 3 for follow up. The caliber of the basilar artery (BA) was measured, as previously described (the midpoint of the basilar artery, and 0.5 cm above and below), in a blinded manner using ImageJ (National Institutes of Health, Bethesda, MD, USA) [1,33]. To assess the degree of DCVS, the relative change between baseline and follow up was compared [1,30,34]. Following baseline DSA on day 0, either induction of SAH or sham procedure was performed, as described earlier [30–32,35,36]. In all animals, intracranial pressure (ICP), arterial blood pressure, and respiration rate were continuously monitored. An ICP probe (Codman Disposable ICP Kit, Spreitenbach, Switzerland) was inserted through a right frontal osteotomy [37]. Arterial blood gas analysis was performed prior to angiography (ABL 725, Radiometer, Copenhagen, Denmark). In prone position, a 27 G spinal access needle was inserted into the cisterna magna. In animals assigned to the SAH, the needle was connected to the catheterized subclavian artery to induce a hemorrhage [30,31]. Sham-operated animals underwent puncture of the cisterna magna, CSF sampling (1.5 mL), and CSF replacement with 1.5 mL artificial CSF (ACSF, Tocris Bioscience, Bristol, UK).

2.3. Blood and CSF Samples Analysis

CSF and blood samples were taken at day 0 and day 3. At day 0, 1.5 mL CSF was aspirated after puncture. The blood samples were collected together with the blood gas analysis using EDTA-coated tubes. The samples were centrifuged with 1500× g for 15 min at 4 °C. The supernatant was segregated and stored at −80 °C until measurement. For IL-1α quantification, a specific IL-1α enzyme-linked immunosorbent assay (ELISA) kit was used (Cayman Chemical, 1180 E. Ellsworth Rd, Ann Arbor, MI, USA). ELISA was performed according to the manufacturers' protocol. Euthanasia was performed on day 3 by injection of 40 mg/kg sodium thiopental (Pentothal, Ospedalia, Hünenberg, Switzerland).

2.4. Statistical Analysis

Data were analyzed and visualized using IBM SPSS statistical software version 21.0 (IBM Corp., New York, NY, USA). Continuous values were given as mean ± SD, if not otherwise indicated. The comparison of baseline and follow up was compared by the Wilcoxson signed rank test (nonparametric, repeated measures). The differences between the normally distributed IL-1α measures and baseline values of two groups and the neurological scores were analyzed by Student's t-test. A p-value < 0.05 was regarded as statistically significant. Correlations were calculated by the Pearson's correlation test.

2.5. Ethic Approval

The study was performed in accordance with the local guidelines for the care and use of experimental animals. The project was performed according to the Animal Research: Reporting of In Vivo Experiments (ARRIVE) guidelines [38] and was performed in accordance with the National Institutes of Health Guidelines for the care and use of experimental animals and with the approval of the Animal Care Committee of the Canton Bern, Switzerland (Approval Nr. BE58/17). A power analysis was not applicable because of the exploratory nature of the study and because it was part of a subproject of a larger study.

3. Results

3.1. Physiological Parameters, ICP Time Course, and SAH and Clinical Scores

A total of 14 (10 in the SAH and four in the sham group) out of 17 rabbits reached the primary endpoint. One rabbit was prematurely excluded after it died before the start of the group-specific procedures. In two rabbits, premature euthanasia was performed due to a severe postoperative neurological deficit after SAH induction. Arterial blood gas analysis was invalid for one animal in each of the SAH and sham operated group during follow up. There were no complications either related to wound healing, cerebrospinal fluid leakage, or infections along the frontal osteotomy sites, subclavian skin incision, or nuchal cisterna injection point.

Arterial blood gas values and basic physiological parameters were within a normal range and there was no significant difference between the groups at baseline and follow up, except for potassium levels which were significantly higher at follow up in the sham operated group (Table 1).

All animals in the SAH group showed a significantly marked ICP increase during SAH induction from baseline to peak ($p = 0.00009$), with a corresponding decrease of cerebral perfusion pressure (CPP) ($p = 0.00089$) (Figure 1, panel left). During SAH induction, there were no significant changes of middle arterial pressure (MAP) and respiratory rate (RR) between the baseline and the peak. There was a trend of worse neurological outcomes during the postsurgical period in the SAH group without significant differences, $p = 0.27$ (Figure 1, panel right).

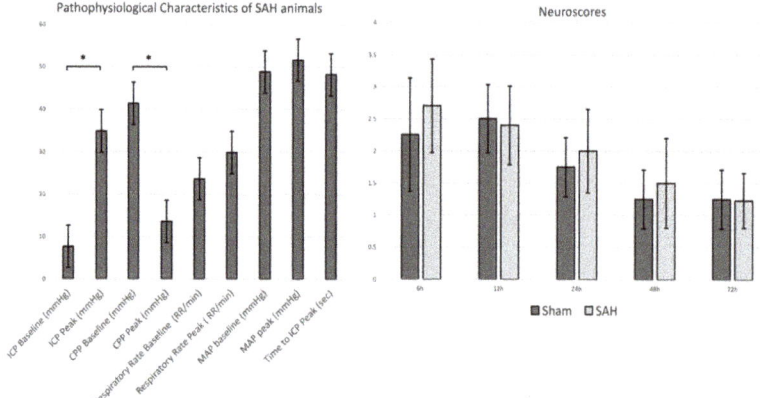

Figure 1. Pathophysiological characteristics of SAH animals (left panel) representing the changes of intracranial pressure (ICP), cerebral perfusion pressure (CPP), respiratory rate, and middle arterial pressure (MAP) at baseline (before SAH induction) and at peak (after SAH induction). Note, between baseline and peak there was a statistically significant increase of ICP and decrease of CPP, respectively. Data are presented as mean ± SD, *: $p < 0.05$. The right panel shows the neuroscores of the rabbits assessed at 6, 12, 24, 48, and 72 h after the surgical interventions. The SAH animals showed a tendency of worse neurological scores as compared to rabbits in the sham group ($p = 0.27$).

All surviving rabbits in the SAH group demonstrated extensive coagulated diffuse subarachnoid blood which resulted in moderate grades of SAH with a mean bleeding sum score [34] of 5.9 (±2.1) in the SAH group as compared to none in the sham group ($p = 0.00002$).

Table 1. Baseline and follow-up analyses for the subarachnoid hemorrhage (SAH) and sham groups.

Parameters	SAH Group ($n = 10$)	Sham Group ($n = 4$)	p-Value
Baseline			
pH	7.3 (±0.1)	7.3 (±0.1)	0.310
pCO_2 (mmHg)	77.1 (±12.5)	70.5 (±14.5)	0.215
pO_2 (mmHg)	340.5 (±95.2)	308 (±150.6)	0.330
HCO_2-mmol/L	28.9 (±7.1)	30.0 (±0.6)	0.325
BE mmol/L	10.8 (±5.9)	9.1 (±2.9)	0.301
SO_2%	99.8 (±0.5)	99.5 (±0.7)	0.268
ctHb (g/dL)	12.3 (±5.3)	12.5 (±0.1)	0.323
Na^+ mmol/L	143.3 (±2.2)	142 (±2.2)	0.164
K^+ mmol/L	3.5 (±0.3)	3.47 (±2.2)	0.401
Ca^{2+} mmol/L	1.6 (±0.1)	1.5 (±0.1)	0.187
Glu mmol/L	15.8 (±3.4)	15.7 (±1.1)	0.487
Lac mmol/L	0.5 (±0.3)	0.5 (±0.1)	0.371
Heart rate/min	187.6 (±18.6)	175.7 (±3.8)	0.223
Middle Arterial Pressure	54.6 (±4.6)	63.7 (±0.3)	0.082
Weight Kg	3.73 (±0.3)	3.53 (±0.2)	0.183
Follow up	SAH Group ($n = 9$)	Sham Group ($n = 3$)	p-Value
pH	7.3 (±0.1)	7.3 (±0.1)	0.349
pCO_2 (mmHg)	70 (±14.3)	68.9 (±14.7)	0.457
pO_2 (mmHg)	351 (±27.8)	431.3 (±29)	0.078
HCO_2-mmol/L	13.2 (±6.2)	22.5 (±7.2)	0.138
BE mmol/L	7.3 (±7.2)	14 (±7.3)	0.186
SO_2%	99.2 (±0.8)	99.5 (±0.7)	0.338
ctHb (g/dL)	10.8 (±0.8)	10.8 (±0.4)	0.50
Na^+ mmol/L	142.7 (±3.8)	143 (±3.5)	0.435
K^+ mmol/L	3.5 (±1.7)	3.9 (±1.5)	0.006
Ca^{2+} mmol/L	1.5 (±0.1)	1.5 (±0.1)	0.449
Glu mmol/L	18.8 (±4.1)	18.6 (±0.4)	0.428
Lac mmol/L	0.6 (±0.1)	0.6 (±0.2)	0.415
Heart rate/min	177.5 (±20.2)	184.5 (±7.5)	0.371
Middle Arterial Pressure	53 (±12.7)	57 (±12.7)	0.399
Weight Kg	3.52 (±0.4)	3.35 (±0.1)	0.07

Baseline and follow-up arterial blood gas analyses, middle arterial pressure, and weight in the SAH and sham groups (Legend: BE, base Excess; ctHb, concentration of hemoglobin; Glu, glucose, and Lac, lactate). Data are presented as mean ± SD.

3.2. Angiographic Delayed Cerebral Vasospasm

At day zero, the baseline angiography in the SAH group showed a mean BA diameter of 310 (±50) μm. At follow up, measurements showed a significantly decreased diameter with a mean of 220 (±60) μm, $p = 0.0001$. The sham group showed a mean BA diameter of 410 (±60) μm at baseline and 450 (±70) μm at follow up ($p = 0.446$), Figure 2.

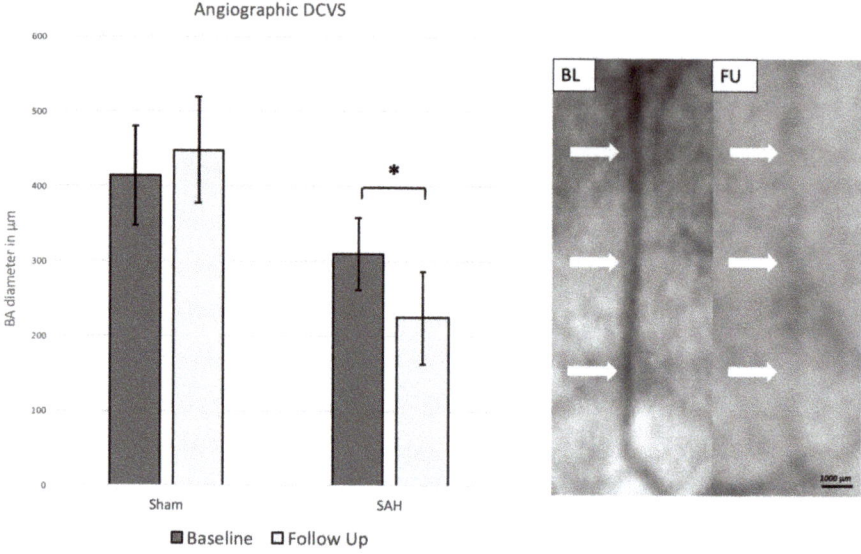

Figure 2. Left: Angiographic mean basilar artery diameter in μm at baseline and follow up. The mean basilar artery diameter decreased significantly at follow up in the SAH group. Data are presented as mean ± SD, *: $p < 0.05$. Right: DSA at baseline (BL) and follow up (FU) demonstrating decrease of caliber size at FU. White arrows: Point of measurement of basilar artery caliber showing decrease of size of the basilar artery at FU.

3.3. CSF and Systemic IL-1α Levels

Notably, overall CSF IL-1α values were significantly higher than serum IL-1α values ($p < 0.0001$). Therefore, we measured CSF IL-1α levels in the range of 5–25 pcg/mL in the CSF while levels in serum were below 1 pcg/mL (Figure 3). In the SAH group, there was a trend of higher CSF IL-1α levels at baseline and follow up as compared with the sham group without statistical significance (Figure 3). In the serum, there was a trend of increasing IL-1α levels between baseline and follow up in the SAH group. When comparing the follow-up values in the sham and SAH groups there was a significant increase of systemic IL-1α in the SAH group as compared with the sham group ($p = 0.042$). The CSF-IL-1α values showed a trend of a negative correlation (Pearson's $r = -0.25$, $p = 0.410$) with the angiographic diameter of the basilar artery. No significant correlation between serum IL-1α values and DCVS could be found (Pearson's $r = -0.03$, $p = 0.856$).

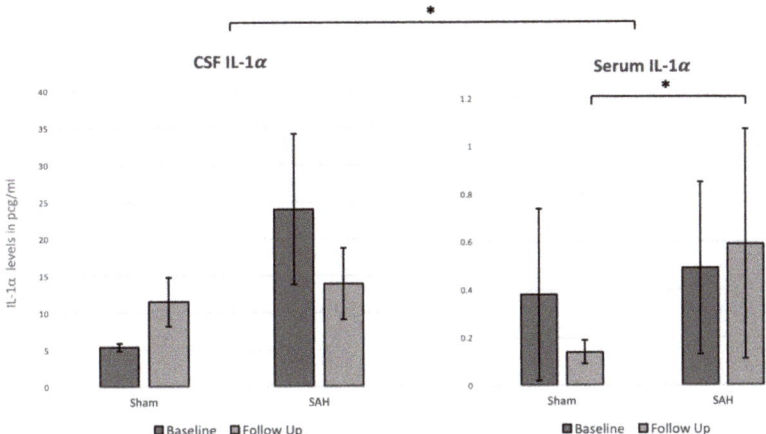

Figure 3. Mean baseline and follow-up IL-1α cerebrospinal fluid (CSF) and serum levels in pcg/mL. Note that the overall CSF IL-1α values were significantly higher as compared to the serum IL-1α levels. Moreover, the serum levels at follow up were significantly higher in the SAH group as compared to the sham group. Data are presented as mean ± SD, *: $p < 0.05$.

4. Discussion

The results of this study demonstrated that SAH was well induced with a significant increase of ICP and a decrease of CPP. DCVS was significantly present in the SAH group. The CSF IL-1α values were overall significantly higher than serum IL-1α values. Moreover, at follow up, the SAH group showed a significantly higher level of IL-1α in serum. A correlation trend between CSF IL-1α and DCVS was found.

Currently, there are neither prophylactic nor therapeutic approaches with convincing efficacy for the treatment and prevention of DCVS and DCI after SAH. Despite various studies confirming the importance of inflammation in the pathophysiology of DCVS and DCI after SAH [1,3,4,23], the clear pathophysiology of the latter remains obscure. This is evident in the role of the different cytokines in the inflammation process and the related effects on neuronal cell death and on endothelial cells, which remain unclear. With this experimental study, we aimed to analyze the behavior of IL-1α in a rabbit closed cranium SAH model. The systemic and CSF IL-1α changes have never been described in a rabbit closed cranium SAH model.

In an ischemic stroke rat model, IL-1α, but not IL-1β, was expressed early on microglia-like cells in the ischemic hemisphere [24,26]. Moreover, IL-1α expression was closely associated with areas of focal blood–brain barrier breakdown and neuronal death, mostly near the penumbra surrounding the infarct, and therefore suggests that IL-1α is the major form of IL-1 contributing to inflammation early after cerebral ischemia [26]. In the context of SAH, a rat SAH model showed that haem induced the expression of IL-1α, produced by microglia and macrophages in the central nervous system, was present early after SAH throughout the brain [23–27,39]. Moreover pharmaceutically synthetized IL-1 Ra showed already promising anti-inflammatory effects in clinical trials of acute stroke and SAH [40,41]. Phase I and phase II clinical randomized trial studies showed that a reduction of IL-6 in serum and CSF and C-reactive protein in a SAH patient treated with an IL-1Ra, however, these studies were not sufficiently powered to analyze the clinical outcome of the patients [41,42]. Our results in this study showed that SAH was well simulated in all the rabbits in the SAH group with a significant increase of ICP and a decrease of CPP, and with a relevant presence of blood in the basal cistern and a significant presence of DCVS at follow up. These results are concordant with our previous studies, confirming the efficacy of the rabbit closed cranium SAH model simulating an aneurysmal SAH [1,30,31].

A correlation trend of CSF IL-1α, but not for serum IL-1α, with DCVS was found. Moreover, the level of systemic IL-1α were significantly higher at follow up in the SAH as compared with the sham group. The overall CSF IL-1α values were found to be higher than the serum values in both groups. This might be explained by a compartmental reaction in the CSF, with IL-1α release, possibly caused either by the surgical procedure itself or due to the generated SAH. Due to the compartmental inflammation reaction after SAH, CSF IL-1α might be more related to the development of DCVS than the serum IL-1α values (especially considering the higher levels of IL-1α in CSF than serum). The fact that serum IL-1α were higher in the SAH group at follow up, without showing a correlation with DCVS, might reflect the compartmental inflammation reaction happening in the CNS.

The results of this study were somewhat inconclusive, especially considering that we did not find any significant CSF increases of IL-1α in the SAH group between baseline and follow up, but only a correlation trend for DCVS. Those results might possibly be explained by the rather small sample size and the lack of power of the study, as this data were extrapolated from one larger study. We should also consider that IL-1α is a generic inflammation cytokine at the top of the inflammation cascade and that other cytokines, like IL-6 which triggers local inflammation and activation of the systemic acute phase response, might play an ever more specific role in the development of DCVS and DCI, as previously described [1,3,4]. Moreover, ELISA quantitative analysis of IL-1α were performed at day zero and day three after induction of SAH. Considering that IL-1α is an early expressed cytokine, possible measurement at day one and day two after SAH induction would have resulted in different values. Further experimental and clinical studies are surely warranted to better understand the behavior of IL-1α in the pathophysiology of DCVS and DCI and its relationship with neuronal cell death and interaction with other cytokines.

5. Conclusions

CSF IL-1α shows that a correlation trend with DCVS and systemic IL-1α is significantly elevated after SAH induction in a rabbit SAH model. IL-1α plays an important role at the beginning of the inflammation cascade in a rabbit closed cranium SAH model.

Author Contributions: D.M.C. and S.M.: design of the study, surgical procedures, collection of data, and drafting of manuscript. S.W., B.E.G., F.S. and S.S.: surgical procedures, collection data, ELISA quantifications. H.R.W. and S.D.S.: collection data, ELISA quantifications. D.C.: anesthesia and monitoring of the rabbits and animal care. All the authors: revision of final manuscript.

Funding: This research was funded by the European Association of Neurological Surgeons (EANS) research grant; from the research fund of the Department of Neurosurgery Kantonsspital Aarau, Switzerland; the HANELA Foundation, Switzerland; and the research fund of the Department of Neurosurgery, University Hospital Basel. The authors have no financial or other conflict of interest to declare.

Acknowledgments: We are deeply grateful to the team of Hans-Ruedi Widmer, PhD at the Neurosurgical Research Institute, the Department of Neurosurgery, University and University Hospital of Bern, Switzerland, for their assistance in ELISA quantifications. We thank the team of the Experimental Surgical Facility and the Central Animal Facility, Department of Biomedical Research, University of Bern, for animal care, anesthesia, and perioperative assistance.

Conflicts of Interest: The authors have no financial or other conflict of interest to declare.

References

1. Croci, D.; Nevzati, E.; Danura, H.; Schöpf, S.; Fandino, J.; Marbacher, S.; Muroi, C. The relationship between IL-6, ET-1 and cerebral vasospasm, in experimental rabbit subarachnoid hemorrhage. *J. Neurosurg. Sci.* **2016**, *63*, 245–250. [CrossRef] [PubMed]
2. Niwa, A.; Osuka, K.; Nakura, T.; Matsuo, N.; Watabe, T.; Takayasu, M. Interleukin-6, MCP-1, IP-10, and MIG are sequentially expressed in cerebrospinal fluid after subarachnoid hemorrhage. *J. Neuroinflamm.* **2017**, *13*, 217. [CrossRef] [PubMed]
3. Fassbender, K.; Hodapp, B.; Rossol, S.; Bertsch, T.; Schmeck, J.; Schütt, S.; Fritzinger, M.; Horn, P.; Vajkoczy, P.; Kreisel, S.; et al. Inflammatory cytokines in subarachnoid haemorrhage: Association with abnormal blood flow velocities in basal cerebral arteries. *J. Neurol. Neurosurg. Psychiatry* **2001**, *70*, 534–537. [CrossRef] [PubMed]

4. Osuka, K.; Suzuki, Y.; Tanazawa, T.; Hattori, K.; Yamamoto, N.; Takayasu, M.; Shibuya, M.; Yoshida, J. Interleukin-6 and development of vasospasm after subarachnoid haemorrhage. *Acta Neurochir. (Wien.)* **1998**, *140*, 943–951. [CrossRef] [PubMed]
5. Dinarello, C.A. A clinical perspective of IL-1β as the gatekeeper of inflammation. *Eur. J. Immunol.* **2011**, *41*, 1203–1217. [CrossRef] [PubMed]
6. Dinarello, C.A. Interleukin-1 in the pathogenesis and treatment of inflammatory diseases. *Blood* **2011**, *117*, 3720–3732. [CrossRef] [PubMed]
7. Dinarello, C.A. The biological properties of interleukin-1. *Eur. Cytokine Netw.* **1994**, *5*, 517–531.
8. Arend, W.P.; Malyak, M.; Guthridge, C.J.; Gabay, C. Interleukin-1 receptor antagonist: Role in biology. *Annu. Rev. Immunol.* **1998**, *16*, 27–55. [CrossRef]
9. Kohno, K.; Kurimoto, M. Interleukin 18, a cytokine which resembles IL-1 structurally and IL-12 functionally but exerts its effect independently of both. *Clin. Immunol. Immunopathol.* **1998**, *86*, 11–15. [CrossRef]
10. Mandrup-Poulsen, T. The role of interleukin-1 in the pathogenesis of IDDM. *Diabetologia* **1996**, *39*, 1005–1029. [CrossRef]
11. Hansen, M.K.; Taishi, P.; Chen, Z.; Krueger, J.M. Vagotomy blocks the induction of interleukin-1beta (IL-1beta) mRNA in the brain of rats in response to systemic IL-1beta. *J. Neurosci.* **1998**, *18*, 2247–2253. [CrossRef] [PubMed]
12. Goehler, L.E.; Relton, J.K.; Dripps, D.; Kiechle, R.; Tartaglia, N.; Maier, S.F.; Watkins, L.R. Vagal paraganglia bind biotinylated interleukin-1 receptor antagonist: A possible mechanism for immune-to-brain communication. *Brain Res. Bull.* **1997**, *43*, 357–364. [CrossRef]
13. Zheng, H.; Fletcher, D.; Kozak, W.; Jiang, M.; Hofmann, K.J.; Conn, C.A.; Soszynski, D.; Grabiec, C.; Trumbauer, M.E.; Shaw, A. Resistance to fever induction and impaired acute-phase response in interleukin-1 beta-deficient mice. *Immunity* **1995**, *3*, 9–19. [CrossRef]
14. Shadiack, A.M.; Hart, R.P.; Carlson, C.D.; Jonakait, G.M. Interleukin-1 induces substance P in sympathetic ganglia through the induction of leukemia inhibitory factor (LIF). *J. Neurosci.* **1993**, *13*, 2601–2609. [CrossRef] [PubMed]
15. Allan, S.M.; Tyrrell, P.J.; Rothwell, N.J. Interleukin-1 and neuronal injury. *Nat. Rev. Immunol.* **2005**, *5*, 629–640. [CrossRef] [PubMed]
16. Allan, S.M. Pragmatic target discovery from novel gene to functionally defined drug target: The interleukin-1 story. *Methods Mol. Med.* **2005**, *104*, 333–346.
17. Kandere-Grzybowska, K.; Letourneau, R.; Kempuraj, D.; Donelan, J.; Poplawski, S.; Boucher, W.; Athanassiou, A.; Theoharides, T.C. IL-1 induces vesicular secretion of IL-6 without degranulation from human mast cells. *J. Immunol.* **2003**, *171*, 4830–4836. [CrossRef]
18. Pluta, R.M.; Hansen-Schwartz, J.; Dreier, J.; Vajkoczy, P.; Macdonald, R.L.; Nishizawa, S.; Kasuya, H.; Wellman, G.; Keller, E.; Zauner, A.; et al. Cerebral vasospasm following subarachnoid hemorrhage: Time for a new world of thought. *Neurol. Res.* **2009**, *31*, 151–158. [CrossRef]
19. Hasan, D.; Chalouhi, N.; Jabbour, P.; Hashimoto, T. Macrophage imbalance (M1 vs. M2) and upregulation of mast cells in wall of ruptured human cerebral aneurysms: Preliminary results. *J. Neuroinflamm.* **2012**, *9*, 222–227. [CrossRef]
20. Korherr, C.; Hofmeister, R.; Wesche, H.; Falk, W. A critical role for interleukin-1 receptor accessory protein in interleukin-1 signaling. *Eur. J. Immunol.* **1997**, *27*, 262–267. [CrossRef]
21. Mosley, B.; Urdal, D.L.; Prickett, K.S.; Larsen, A.; Cosman, D.; Conlon, P.J.; Gillis, S.; Dower, S.K. The interleukin-1 receptor binds the human interleukin-1 alpha precursor but not the interleukin-1 beta precursor. *J. Biol. Chem.* **1987**, *262*, 2941–2944.
22. Hannum, C.H.; Wilcox, C.J.; Arend, W.P.; Joslin, F.G.; Dripps, D.J.; Heimdal, P.L.; Armes, L.G.; Sommer, A.; Eisenberg, S.P.; Thompson, R.C. Interleukin-1 receptor antagonist activity of a human interleukin-1 inhibitor. *Nature* **1990**, *343*, 336–340. [CrossRef]
23. Greenhalgh, A.D.; Brough, D.; Robinson, E.M.; Girard, S.; Rothwell, N.J.; Allan, S.M. Interleukin-1 receptor antagonist is beneficial after subarachnoid haemorrhage in rat by blocking haem-driven inflammatory pathology. *Dis. Model. Mech.* **2012**, *5*, 823–833. [CrossRef] [PubMed]
24. Brough, D.; Dénes, Á. Interleukin-1α and brain inflammation. *IUBMB Life* **2015**, *67*, 323–330. [CrossRef]
25. Orsini, F.; Fumagalli, S.; Császár, E.; Tóth, K.; De Blasio, D.; Zangari, R.; Lénárt, N.; Dénes, Á.; De Simoni, M.-G. Mannose-Binding Lectin Drives Platelet Inflammatory Phenotype and Vascular Damage After Cerebral Ischemia in Mice via IL (Interleukin)-1α. *Arterioscler. Thromb. Vasc. Biol.* **2018**, *38*, 2678–2690. [CrossRef]

26. Luheshi, N.M.; Kovács, K.J.; Lopez-Castejon, G.; Brough, D.; Dénes, Á. Interleukin-1α expression precedes IL-1β after ischemic brain injury and is localised to areas of focal neuronal loss and penumbral tissues. *J. Neuroinflamm.* **2011**, *8*, 186. [CrossRef]
27. Eisenhut, M. Vasospasm in cerebral inflammation. *Int. J. Inflam.* **2014**, *2014*, 509707–509714. [CrossRef]
28. Randomisation and online databases for clinical trials. Available online: https://www.sealedenvelope.com/ (accessed on 5 March 2018).
29. Endo, S.; Branson, P.J.; Alksne, J.F. Experimental model of symptomatic vasospasm in rabbits. *Stroke* **1988**, *19*, 1420–1425. [CrossRef] [PubMed]
30. Marbacher, S.; Nevzati, E.; Croci, D.; Erhardt, S.; Muroi, C.; Jakob, S.M.; Fandino, J. The rabbit shunt model of subarachnoid haemorrhage. *Transl. Stroke Res.* **2014**, *5*, 669–680. [CrossRef] [PubMed]
31. Andereggen, L.; Neuschmelting, V.; von Gunten, M.; Widmer, H.R.; Takala, J.; Jakob, S.M.; Fandino, J.; Marbacher, S. The rabbit blood-shunt model for the study of acute and late sequelae of subarachnoid hemorrhage: Technical aspects. *J. Vis. Exp.* **2014**, *92*, e52132. [CrossRef]
32. Marbacher, S.; Fathi, A.-R.; Muroi, C.; Coluccia, D.; Andereggen, L.; Neuschmelting, V.; Widmer, H.R.; Jakob, S.M.; Fandino, J. The rabbit blood shunt subarachnoid haemorrhage model. *Acta Neurochir. Suppl.* **2015**, *120*, 337–342. [PubMed]
33. Zhang, Z.-W.; Yanamoto, H.; Nagata, I.; Miyamoto, S.; Nakajo, Y.; Xue, J.-H.; Iihara, K.; Kikuchi, H. Platelet-derived growth factor-induced severe and chronic vasoconstriction of cerebral arteries: Proposed growth factor explanation of cerebral vasospasm. *Neurosurgery* **2010**, *66*, 728–735. [CrossRef] [PubMed]
34. Marbacher, S.; Neuschmelting, V.; Andereggen, L.; Widmer, H.R.; von Gunten, M.; Takala, J.; Jakob, S.M.; Fandino, J. Early brain injury linearly correlates with reduction in cerebral perfusion pressure during the hyperacute phase of subarachnoid hemorrhage. *Intensive Care Med. Exp.* **2014**, *2*, 30. [CrossRef] [PubMed]
35. Marbacher, S.; Sherif, C.; Neuschmelting, V.; Schläppi, J.-A.; Takala, J.; Jakob, S.M.; Fandino, J. Extra-intracranial blood shunt mimicking aneurysm rupture: Intracranial-pressure-controlled rabbit subarachnoid hemorrhage model. *J. Neurosci. Methods* **2010**, *191*, 227–233. [CrossRef] [PubMed]
36. Marbacher, S.; Andereggen, L.; Neuschmelting, V.; Widmer, H.R.; von Gunten, M.; Takala, J.; Jakob, S.M.; Fandino, J. A new rabbit model for the study of early brain injury after subarachnoid hemorrhage. *J. Neurosci. Methods* **2012**, *208*, 138–145. [CrossRef]
37. Marbacher, S.; Milavec, H.; Neuschmelting, V.; Andereggen, L.; Erhardt, S.; Fandino, J. Outer skull landmark-based coordinates for measurement of cerebral blood flow and intracranial pressure in rabbits. *J. Neurosci. Methods* **2011**, *201*, 322–326. [CrossRef] [PubMed]
38. NC3Rs Reporting Guidelines Working Group. Animal research: Reporting in vivo experiments: The ARRIVE guidelines. *J. Physiol. (Lond.)* **2010**, *588*, 2519–2521. [CrossRef]
39. Zheng, Y.; Humphry, M.; Maguire, J.J.; Bennett, M.R.; Clarke, M.C.H. Intracellular interleukin-1 receptor 2 binding prevents cleavage and activity of interleukin-1α, controlling necrosis-induced sterile inflammation. *Immunity* **2013**, *38*, 285–295. [CrossRef]
40. Emsley, H.C.A.; Smith, C.J.; Georgiou, R.F.; Vail, A.; Hopkins, S.J.; Rothwell, N.J.; Tyrrell, P.J. Acute Stroke Investigators A randomised phase II study of interleukin-1 receptor antagonist in acute stroke patients. *J. Neurol. Neurosurg. Psychiatry* **2005**, *76*, 1366–1372. [CrossRef]
41. Galea, J.; Ogungbenro, K.; Hulme, S.; Patel, H.; Scarth, S.; Hoadley, M.; Illingworth, K.; McMahon, C.J.; Tzerakis, N.; King, A.T.; et al. Reduction of inflammation after administration of interleukin-1 receptor antagonist following aneurysmal subarachnoid hemorrhage: Results of the Subcutaneous Interleukin-1Ra in SAH (SCIL-SAH) study. *J. Neurosurg.* **2018**, *128*, 515–523. [CrossRef]
42. Singh, N.; Hopkins, S.J.; Hulme, S.; Galea, J.P.; Hoadley, M.; Vail, A.; Hutchinson, P.J.; Grainger, S.; Rothwell, N.J.; King, A.T.; et al. The effect of intravenous interleukin-1 receptor antagonist on inflammatory mediators in cerebrospinal fluid after subarachnoid haemorrhage: A phase II randomised controlled trial. *J. Neuroinflamm.* **2014**, *11*, 1. [CrossRef] [PubMed]

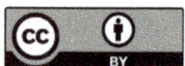

© 2019 by the authors. Licensee MDPI, Basel, Switzerland. This article is an open access article distributed under the terms and conditions of the Creative Commons Attribution (CC BY) license (http://creativecommons.org/licenses/by/4.0/).

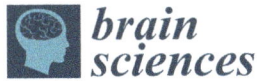

Review

The Role of Sartans in the Treatment of Stroke and Subarachnoid Hemorrhage: A Narrative Review of Preclinical and Clinical Studies

Stefan Wanderer [1,2,*], Basil E. Grüter [1,2], Fabio Strange [1,2], Sivani Sivanrupan [2], Stefano Di Santo [3], Hans Rudolf Widmer [3], Javier Fandino [1,2], Serge Marbacher [1,2] and Lukas Andereggen [1,2]

[1] Department of Neurosurgery, Kantonsspital Aarau, 5001 Aarau, Switzerland; basil.grueter@ksa.ch (B.E.G.); fabio.strange@ksa.ch (F.S.); javier.fandino@ksa.ch (J.F.); serge.marbacher@ksa.ch (S.M.); lukas.andereggen@ksa.ch (L.A.)
[2] Cerebrovascular Research Group, Neurosurgery, Department of BioMedical Research, University of Bern, 3008 Bern, Switzerland; sivani.sivanrupan@students.unibe.ch
[3] Department of Neurosurgery, Neurocenter and Regenerative Neuroscience Cluster, Inselspital, Bern University Hospital, University of Bern, 3010 Bern, Switzerland; stefano.disanto@insel.ch (S.D.S.); hansrudolf.widmer@insel.ch (H.R.W.)
* Correspondence: stefan.wanderer@ksa.ch or neurosurgery@ksa.ch; Tel.: +41-628-384-141

Received: 17 January 2020; Accepted: 5 March 2020; Published: 7 March 2020

Abstract: *Background*: Delayed cerebral vasospasm (DCVS) due to aneurysmal subarachnoid hemorrhage (aSAH) and its sequela, delayed cerebral ischemia (DCI), are associated with poor functional outcome. Endothelin-1 (ET-1) is known to play a major role in mediating cerebral vasoconstriction. Angiotensin-II-type-1-receptor antagonists such as Sartans may have a beneficial effect after aSAH by reducing DCVS due to crosstalk with the endothelin system. In this review, we discuss the role of Sartans in the treatment of stroke and their potential impact in aSAH. *Methods*: We conducted a literature research of the MEDLINE PubMed database in accordance with PRISMA criteria on articles published between 1980 to 2019 reviewing: "Sartans AND ischemic stroke". Of 227 studies, 64 preclinical and 19 clinical trials fulfilled the eligibility criteria. *Results*: There was a positive effect of Sartans on ischemic stroke in both preclinical and clinical settings (attenuating ischemic brain damage, reducing cerebral inflammation and infarct size, increasing cerebral blood flow). In addition, Sartans reduced DCVS after aSAH in animal models by diminishing the effect of ET-1 mediated vasoconstriction (including cerebral inflammation and cerebral epileptogenic activity reduction, cerebral blood flow autoregulation restoration as well as pressure-dependent cerebral vasoconstriction). *Conclusion*: Thus, Sartans might play a key role in the treatment of patients with aSAH.

Keywords: aneurysmal subarachnoid hemorrhage; delayed cerebral vasospasm; ischemic stroke; Sartans; therapeutic interventions

---

1. Introduction

Aneurysmal subarachnoid hemorrhage (aSAH) induces delayed cerebral vasospasm (DCVS) [1], cerebral inflammation [2,3], early brain injury [4], cortical spreading depression [5], delayed cerebral ischemia (DCI) [6], and lack of cerebral autoregulation [7] contributing to poor functional patients' outcome. DCVS remains a major cause of patient's morbidity and mortality by inducing delayed cerebral ischemia [8].

Multiple studies showed that endothelin-1 (ET-1), a most potent vasoconstrictor [9–11], plays a key role in the development of DCVS [12–19]. Although endothelin-A-receptor (ET_A-R) antagonists in the treatment of DCVS in animal models are effective [10,20], clinical studies did not show beneficial effects [21,22]. It has been reported that the polypeptide angiotensin-II acts through two specific receptors, in essence the angiotensin-II-type-1- and angiotensin-II-type-2-receptor (AT_2-1-R and AT_2-2-R). Important to note is that activation of the AT_2-1-R results in vasoconstriction while binding of angiotensin-II to the AT_2-2-R causes vasorelaxation [23]. In line with this notion, preclinical as well as clinical trials showed promising results of Sartans, which are AT_2-1-R antagonists, in ischemic stroke. Hence, Sartans may have a positive effect after aSAH by reducing DCVS due to crosstalk with the endothelin system. Thus, we aimed to analyze the potential role of Sartans in the treatment of aSAH.

2. Materials and Methods

We conducted a systematic literature research of the MEDLINE PubMed database in accordance with PRISMA guidelines on preclinical studies on the one and on clinical studies on the other hand published between 1980 to 2019 reviewing: "Sartans and ischemic stroke" [24]. Only articles in English were chosen for review. Search items with "Sartans" ($n = 19,064$) and "ischemic stroke" ($n = 89,465$) were extracted. For "Sartans AND ischemic stroke", 227 publications met the inclusion criteria by excluding studies with commentary only, any duplicates, or results not commenting on cerebral effects of Sartans.

Two hundred and twenty-seven studies were assessed for eligibility, 83 met inclusion criteria for systematic review and qualitative analysis with 64 preclinical studies (Figure 1 demonstrates the inclusion pathway for basic research studies selected via MEDLINE PubMed search) and 19 clinical studies (Figure 2 shows the inclusion pathway for clinical research studies selected via MEDLINE PubMed search).

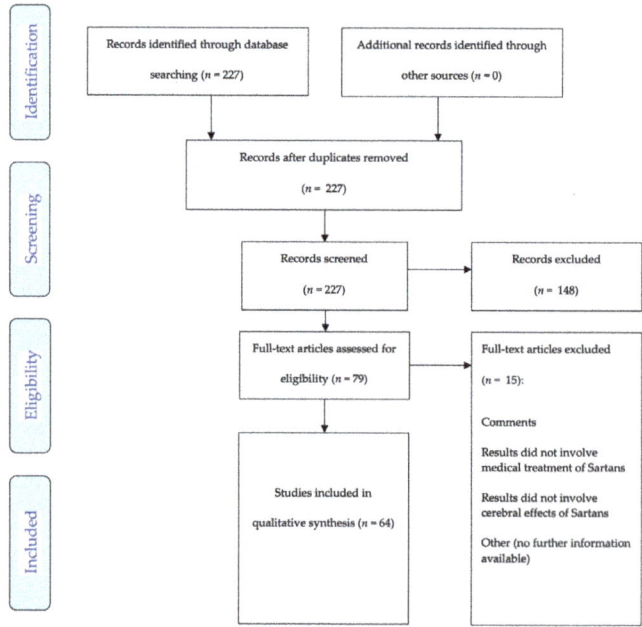

Figure 1. Two hundred and twenty-seven articles (published 01-01-1980–01-07-2019) were detected for preclinical and clinical research articles. After manual abstract screening for preclinical research articles only, 79 articles remained for further analysis. Each of the 79 articles was explicitly screened for potential drug applications after ischemic stroke. Finally, 64 articles were included for qualitative analysis.

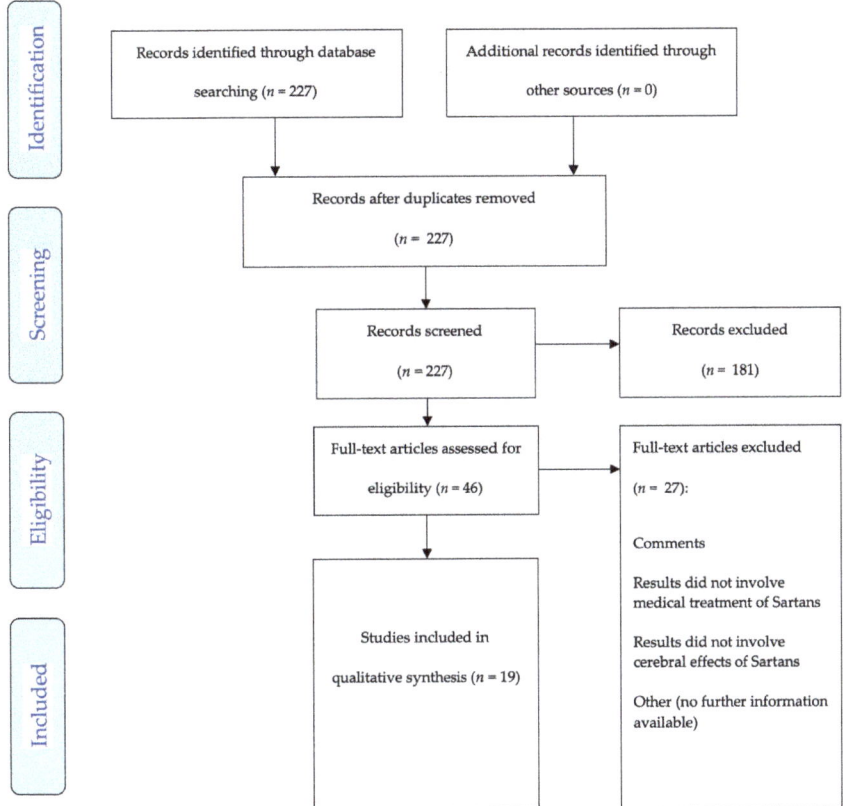

Figure 2. Two hundred and twenty-seven articles (published 01-01-1980–01-07-2019) were detected for preclinical and clinical research articles. After manual abstract screening for clinical research articles only, 46 articles remained for further analysis. Each of the 46 articles was explicitly screened for potential drug applications after ischemic stroke. Finally, 19 articles were included for final analysis.

Of the articles included in the final analysis, a systematic review on the beneficial and non-beneficial effect in the preclinical and clinical settings was performed. Summary measures are reported as outcome measures (i.e., infarct size, neurocognition, inflammation).

3. Results

3.1. Preclinical Studies on Sartans in Animal Models of Ischemic Stroke

The search finally yielded 64 preclinical studies on "Sartans AND ischemic stroke", eligible for systematic review (Table 1).

Table 1. Tabular listing of different preclinical studies showing various effects of Sartan administration (Abbreviations: Angiotensin-II-type-1-receptor (AT$_2$-1-R); Angiotensin-II-type-2-receptor (AT$_2$-2-R); common carotid artery occlusion (CCAO); chemokine receptor 2 (CCR2); cluster of differentiation (CD); candesartan (CS); desoxy ribonucleic acid (DNA); endothelial nitric oxide synthase (eNOS); endothelin-A-receptor (ET$_A$-R); hours (h); inducible nitric oxide synthase (iNOS); irbesartan (IS); kilogram (kg); losartan (LS); middle cerebral artery occlusion (MCAO); matrix-metallo-proteinase (MMP); messenger ribonucleic acid (mRNA); milligram (mg); minutes (min); n-acetyl-glucosamine oligomer (NAGO); nlr family pyrin domain containing 3 (NLRP3); oxygen glucose deprivation (OGD); olmesartan (OMS); stroke-resistant spontaneously hypertensive rats (SR-SHR); telmisartan (TMS); tumor necrosis factor alpha (TNFα); ribonucleic acid (RNA); vascular endothelial growth factor (VEGF); valsartan (VS)).

Drug	Model	Outcome	Beneficial Effect	Special Remarks
TMS [25]	Global ischemic mice model	Cerebral perfusion	Restored cerebral blood flow	-
TMS [26]	MCAO mice	Neuroscore, infarct size	Improved neuroscore and decreased infarct size, increased cerebral blood flow, reduced superoxide production and inflammatory cytokine expression	-
TMS [27]	Murine model of transient and permanent focal ischemia	Infarct size, reperfusion injury	Reduced stroke volume 72 h after transient ischemia, likewise pro-inflammatory adhesion molecules and infiltration of inflammatory cells in the ischemic region	No reduction in stroke volume 72 h after permanent ischemia
TMS [28]	MCAO mice	Focal brain ischemia, atherosclerotic lesions	Attenuated ischemic brain damage, neurological deficits and superoxide production in ischemic area; attenuated reduction of cerebral blood flow in the penumbra without significantly changing blood pressure	Anti-atherosclerotic effects
TMS [29]	MCAO rat	Cerebral perfusion	Improved cerebral blood flow, enhanced vascular density (CD31 immunofluorescence staining), antiapoptotic effects	-
TMS [30]	MCAO rat	Cognitive function, level of matrix metalloproteinases	Improved spatial memory ability, decreased expression levels of MMP-2 and MMP-9	-
TMS [31]	MCAO rat	Behavior alterations, neuroprotective effects on secondary reperfusion phase	Normalized behavioral alterations comparable to pre-ischemic treatment (protected neurons from ischemic reperfusion injury), attenuated excitatory amino acid release in secondary reperfusion phase	In combination with nimodipine. Drug treatments immediately after reperfusion, effects compared with pretreatment

Table 1. Cont.

Drug	Model	Outcome	Beneficial Effect	Special Remarks
TMS [32]	MCAO rat	Effects on neurovascular unit and neuroinflammation	Reduced decrease of NAGO-positive endothelium, similar increase of MMP-9 positive neurons and NLRP3-positive inflammasome in the cerebral cortex	Low dose TMS improved changes without lowering blood pressure, high dose TMS further improved changes with lowering blood pressure
TMS [33]	Open skull preparation rat	Cerebral arteriolar pressure, cerebral blood flow, internal vessel diameter	Normalization of arteriolar pressure and lower limit of cerebral autoregulation	Combined with Ramipril
TMS [34]	MCAO rats	Metabolic related post-ischemic changes	Ameliorated metabolic related post-ischemic changes	-
TMS [35]	MCAO rats	Neurological outcome, infarct volume, inflammation	Improved outcome, reduced infarct volume and inflammation	Subcutaneous TMS application 5 days prior to MCAO with reperfusion
TMS [36]	MCAO rats	Infarct volume, immunohistochemical parameters	Significantly reduced infarct volume, reduced neurotoxic cytosolic phospholipase A2, ameliorates ischemic changes of neurons in the peri-infarct area	Pretreatment for 7 days
TMS [37]	Collagenase infusion or autologous blood injection to induce intracerebral hemorrhage in rats	Hemorrhage volume, functional recovery	Reduced hemorrhage volume, brain edema, inflammatory/apoptotic cells in perihematomal area; induced endothelial nitric-oxide-synthase, decreased oxidative stress, apoptotic signals, and TNFα	-
TMS [38]	Stroke-resistant spontaneously hypertensive rats	Oxidative stress	Reduced advanced glycation end product, 4-hydroxy-2-nonenal- and phosphorylated a-synuclein-positive cells in the cerebral cortex and hippocampus	-
CS [39]	MCAO mice	Ischemic brain damage	Reduced ischemic brain area and neurological deficits in non-hypotensive doses; improved reduction of brain surface blood flow and inhibited superoxide production in the cortex and brain arterial wall at non-hypotensive and hypotensive doses; AT_2-2-R expression in the ischemic area was increased by prior pretreatment with CS	-

Table 1. *Cont.*

Drug	Model	Outcome	Beneficial Effect	Special Remarks
CS [40]	MCAO mice	Antioxidant enzyme activity	Restored superoxide dismutase activity and cerebral blood flow	-
CS [41]	MCAO rats	Neurobehavioral outcome, infarct size, vascular density	Improved neurobehavioral outcome, reduced infarct size and vascular density	In vitro vascular density was assessed using human brain endothelial cells
CS [42]	MCAO rats	Infarct size, neurological outcome	Improved neurobehavioral and motor functions, decreased infarct size	Intravenous CS administration
CS [43]	MCAO rats	Neurological outcome	Improved recovery from ischemic stroke	Only 0.3 mg/kg CS with neuroprotective function
CS [44]	MCAO rats	Neurological outcome, oxidative enzymes	Improved motor function and reduced endoplasmatic reticulum stress markers	Only early beneficial effect after 24 h
CS [45]	MCAO rats	Neurological outcome, vascular density/synaptogenesis	Improved functional outcome, increased vascular density/synaptogenesis only in the control group	Intracerebroventricular injection of short hairpin RNA lentiviral particles to knock down brain-derived neurotrophic factor or nontargeting control vector
CS [46]	MCAO rats	Angiogenesis	Induced prolonged proangiogenic effect and upregulation of VEGF-A and VEGF-B; stabilized hypoxia-inducible factor-1a and preserves angiopoetin-1	-
CS [47]	Spontaneously hypertensive rats	Angiogenesis	Exerted proangiogenic effects on brain microvascular endothelial cells	-
CS [48]	In vitro monolayer model using rat brain capillary endothelial cells	Stability of blood brain barrier	Improved cell function and viability of brain capillary endothelial cells under OGD	Normoxia versus 6 h OGD
CS [49]	MCAO rats	Neurological outcome, infarct size	Improved neurological function, significantly reduced blood brain barrier disruption/edema/infarct volume	-
CS [50]	MCAO rats	Infarct size, functional recovery, neuroplasticity	Significantly reduced infarct size, ameliorated functional recovery and increased neuroplasticity markers	-

Table 1. Cont.

Drug	Model	Outcome	Beneficial Effect	Special Remarks
CS [51]	MCAO rats	Infarct size, neurological outcome	Decreased infarct size and improved neurological outcome	-
CS [52]	MCAO rats	Mortality, infarct size	Significantly reduced mortality and infarct size	-
CS [53]	MCAO rats	Infarct size	Reduced infarct size	Oral administration
CS [54]	MCAO rats	Infarct size, edema, neurological outcome	Reduced infarct size, edema formation and improves neurological outcome	-
CS [55]	MCAO rats	Infarct size, neurological outcome	Significantly reduced stroke volume and improved neurological outcome	-
CS [56]	MCAO rats	Infarct size, edema	Reduced infarct size and edema, improved neurologic function	-
CS [57]	MCAO rats	Infarct volume, neurological deficit	Reduced infarct size and improved neurologic outcome	-
CS [58]	MCAO rats	Infarct volume, neurological deficits	Reduced infarct size, improved neurological outcome, reduced lipid peroxidation	Subcutaneous infusion for 14 days
CS [59]	MCAO rats	Infarct size, neurological deficits	Reduced infarct size/edema and improved neurological outcome	Long-term blockade (subcutaneous injection twice daily 5 days before ischemia), not short-term administration (intravenous once 4 h prior to ischemia), improves neurological outcome
CS [60]	MCAO rats	Infarct volume, brain edema	Significantly reduced cortical infarct volume and brain edema	-
CS [61]	Bilateral CCAO rats	Neurological outcome, oxidative damage	Attenuated neurobehavioral alterations, oxidative damage and restored mitochondrial enzyme dysfunction	Occlusion for 30 min, followed by 24 h reperfusion; CS pretreatment for 7 days
CS [62]	MCAO rats	Infarct size	Reduced infarct area	-
CS [63]	MCAO rats	Infarct size, neurological outcome	Pretreatment reduced infarct area and improved neurological outcome	-
CS [64]	MCAO rats	Infarct size, neurological outcome	Reduced infarct size and neurological deficits; significantly reduced mRNA expression of inflammatory markers	-

Table 1. *Cont.*

Drug	Model	Outcome	Beneficial Effect	Special Remarks
CS [65]	Spontaneously hypertensive rats	AT_2-1-R expression	Increased AT_2-2-R expression in spontaneously hypertensive rats	CS application via subcutaneous osmotic minipumps for 4 weeks
CS [66]	MCAO rats	Neurological outcome, vascular density	Improved neurological outcome and increased vascular density	-
CS [67]	Embolic stroke model	Mortality, neurological outcome, infarct size	Significantly decreased mortality, neurological deficits, and infarct size	Injection of calibrated microspheres
CS [68]	MCAO rat	Infarct size, neurological outcome	Reduced infarct size and improved neurological outcome	Combined treatment with ET_A-R antagonist
CS [69]	MCAO rats	Contractile response to angiotensin II	Abolished the enhanced responses to angiotensin II	-
CS [70]	MCAO rats	Infarct volume, neurological outcome	Reduced infarct size with low but not high dose of CS, improved neurological outcome	Subcutaneous CS administration
CS [71]	MCAO rats	Infarct size, neuroscores, cerebral blood flow	Reduced infarct size and increased cerebral blood flow	Intravenous CS administration
CS [72]	Spontaneously hypertensive rats	Vascular remodeling, expression of eNOS/iNOS	Reversed negative vascular remodeling and alterations in eNOS/iNOS expression	-
OMS [73]	Bilateral CCAO mice	Cognitive impairment	Ameliorated cognitive impairment	-
OMS [74]	Single carotid ligation stroke model gerbil	Survival	Significantly increased survival at day 30	-
OMS [75]	MCAO rats	Neurological outcome, infarct size, cell death	Significantly improved functional scores, reduced infarct size and cell death	Only continuous administration of OMS before and after stroke reduced oxidative stress levels
OMS [76]	MCAO rats	Infarct volume	Reduced infarct volume 48 h after transient focal brain ischemia	OMS administration via drinking water
OMS [77]	MCAO rats	Stroke index score, infarct volume, quantity of MMPs	Improved stroke index score, infarct volume, reduced cerebral edema and upregulation of MMPs	-

Table 1. Cont.

Drug	Model	Outcome	Beneficial Effect	Special Remarks
VS [78]	MCAO mice	Infarct volume, DNA damage, superoxide production	Significantly reduced infarct size, DNA damage, superoxide production, mRNA levels of monocyte chemoattractant protein-1, increases cerebral blood flow, increased eNOS activation and nitric oxide production	-
VS [79]	MCAO mice	Infarct volume, neurological outcome	Significantly reduced infarct volume and improved neurological outcome	-
VS [80]	MCAO mice	Infarct volume, neurological outcome	Significantly reduced ischemic area, neurological deficits, reduction of cerebral blood flow and superoxide production	-
VS [81]	High salt loaded SR-SHR	Brain injury	Enhanced protective effects against brain injury, white matter lesions and glial activation	Combined with amlodipine
IS [82]	MCAO rats	Infarct size, neurological outcome	Reduced infarct size and number of apoptotic cells in the peri-infart cortex on day 3, attenuated invasion of microglia and macrophages on day 3 and 7 after ischemia	-
IS [83]	MCAO rats	Neurological outcome	Significantly improved neurological outcome	Administration of IS intracerebroventricularly over 5 days
IS [84]	MCAO rats	Infarct size	Reduced infarct volume	Coadministration of propagermanium (CCR2 antagonist)
LS [85]	Single carotid ligation stroke model gerbil	Mortality	Did not increase mortality after unilateral carotid ligation in gerbils	-
LS [86]	MCAO mice	OGD-induced cell injury	Abolished OGD-induced exaggeration of cell injury in mice overexpressing renin and angiotensinogen animals	-
LS [87]	MCAO rats	Gene expression levels of pro-apoptotic genes	Significant reduced gene expression of pro-apoptotic genes	-
LS [88]	Cerebral focal ischemia by cauterization of cortical surface vessels rats	Cessation of blood flow, infarct size	Maintained angiogenesis, vascular delivery, and significantly decreased infarct size	Administration of LS in drinking water 2 weeks before inducing ischemia

Telmisartan (TMS), a selective AT_2-1-R antagonist, displayed the capacity to increase cerebral blood flow (CBF) in global cerebral ischemia [25]. It ameliorated reduction of CBF in the penumbra (0.3 mg/kg/day) without significant changes in blood pressure (BP) [28]. Following middle cerebral artery occlusion (MCAO), TMS decreased ischemic infarct area, reduced superoxide production and expression of inflammatory cytokines, infiltration of inflammatory cells, improved neurological scores, and increased CBF [26,27]. Angiogenesis in ischemic areas after MCAO was enhanced by TMS, as well as neuroregeneration by downregulating caspase activation [29]. A combination of TMS with nimodipine (2.5–5 mg/kg) in a transient MCAO rat model revealed beneficial influences affecting the attenuation of excitatory amino acids in different brain regions nine days after MCAO with neurobehavioural outcomes normalized seven days after MCAO [31]. Low doses of TMS (0.3–3 mg/kg/d) after MCAO in a model of stroke-resistant spontaneously hypertensive rats (SR-SHR) reduced progressive decrease of N-acetylglucosamine oligomer and increase of MMP-9 positive neurons without reducing BP [32]. Likewise combination therapies with ramipril (0.8 mg/kg per day TMS + 0.1 mg/kg per day ramipril or 0.5 mg/kg per day TMS + 0.25 mg/kg per day ramipril) normalized BP as well as maintained cerebral blood flow autoregulation [33]. Deguchi et al. demonstrated that TMS dose-dependently (0.3 mg/kg/day or 3 mg/kg/day) ameliorated metabolic syndrome related changes in the post stroke brain of SR-SHR with direct neuroprotective effects [34]. Moreover, incidence of stroke was reduced along with prolonged survival and improved neurological outcome following TMS application (0.5 mg/kg once daily) [35]. Pretreatment of rats with TMS (1 mg/kg) seven days before inducing cerebral ischemia also showed significant reduced infarct size and histopathologically normal appearance of neurons in the periinfarct cortical regions [36].

Candesartan (CS), another AT_2-1-R antagonist, reduced ischemic brain damage following MCAO occlusion [39]. CS and curcumin together significantly restored superoxide dismutase activity and blood flow compared with the untreated group [40]. Further, CS upregulated vascular endothelial growth factor (VEGF) B after induction of focal cerebral ischemia using a MCAO model. In contrast to saline-treatment after reperfusion, CS further improved neurobehavioral and motor functions and decreased infarct size [41]. VEGF-B silencing was shown to diminish CS (1 mg/kg) protective effects [42]. CS (0.3 mg/kg) was able to improve recovery from ischemic stroke in low doses by maintaining blood pressure during reperfusion [43]. CS induced early protective effects with improvement in motor function, upregulated brain-derived neutrotrophic factor (BDNF), and also reduced endoplasmatic reticulum stress markers [44]. In a MCAO BDNF, knock-out model rats received CS or saline at reperfusion for 14 days, revealing better functional outcomes, increased vascular density, and synaptogenesis in the CS (1 mg/kg) group [45,46]. In addition, CS (0.16 µM) significantly increased BDNF production [47]. Furthermore, CS (10 nM) improved cell function and viability of brain capillary endothelial cells under oxygen glucose deprivation, providing protective blood–brain-barrier (BBB) effects [48]. In other transient MCAO rat models, CS (0.1 mg/kg; 0.3 mg/kg; 1.5 or 10 mg/kg per day; 0.1, 1 and 10 mg/kg; 0.1, 0.3 or 1 mg/kg; 0.1 mg/kg twice daily; 1 mg/kg; 0.3 or 3 mg/kg per day; 0.5 mg/kg per day for 14 days; 0.1 or 0.3 mg/kg; 0.5 mg/kg per day for 3 to 14 days) showed improved neurological function with significant reduction in BBB disruption, in cerebral ischemia, and in edema [39,49–60]. In a bilateral common carotid artery occlusion (CCAO) model in rats, pretreatment with CS (0.1 and 0.3 mg/kg) and atorvastatin significantly attenuated neurobehavioral alterations, oxidative damage, and restored mitochondrial enzyme dysfunction compared to the control group [61,62]. AT_2-1-R administration prior to ET-1 induced MCAO provides neuroprotective effects, with CS (0.2 mg/kg per day for seven days) pretreatment attenuating infarct size and neurological deficits without altering systemic BP [63]. Pretreatment with CS for five days significantly decreased mortality, neurological deficits, and infarct size [67]. A combined inhibition of AT_2-1- (0.05 mg/kg per day) and ET_A-receptors decreased brain damage as well; additionally, an upregulation of AT_2-1-R in ischemic middle cerebral artery smooth muscle cells (SMCs) was found [68,69]. Also, early (3 h) and delayed (24 h) effects of CS treatment (0.3 and 3 mg/kg) continued for seven days after onset of MCAO with reperfusion in normotensive rats involved a reduction of the infarct volume by low doses of CS [70].

CBF in CS (0.5 mg/kg) pretreated animals at 0.5 h after MCAO was significantly increased compared to the control group [71]. Other groups additionally showed a four-week CS-pretreatment (0.3 mg/kg per day) before MCAO clearly associated with complete reversal of a decreased lumen diameter and increased media thickness as well as decreased endothelial nitric oxide synthase (eNOS) and increased inducible nitric oxide synthase (iNOS) protein and mRNA in SR-SHR and in a normotensive control group [72].

Olmesartan (OMS), an AT_2-1-R antagonist, has been evaluated in a bilateral CCAO model in mice, revealing improved cognitive outcome, neuroprotective effects, attenuation of oxidative hippocampal stress, and suppression of BBB disruption compared to control groups [73]. A single carotid ligation stroke model in gerbils showed that OMS (10 mg/kg per day started 36 h after stroke) was associated with an increased survival [74]. Other studies demonstrated that OMS (10 mg/kg per day for 14 days after infarct; 10 mg/kg per day for 7 days before and 14 days after infarct; 10 mg/kg per day for 7 days before infarct) treatment in a rat MCAO model showed significantly better functional scores and reduced infarct size and cell death [75]. OMS (0.01 or 0.1 µmol/kg per hour for seven days) reduced brain angiotensin II, MMP-2 and MMP-9 upregulation following brain ischemia [77].

Valsartan (VS), a selective AT_2-1-R antagonist, reduced ischemic brain area and improved the neurological deficit after MCAO with restoration of cerebral blood flow [78]. VS significantly reduced infarct volume and improved the neurological deficit scores. VS at nonhypotensive doses significantly diminished ischemic area, neurological deficits, and reduction of cerebral blood flow as well as superoxide production [27,78,80].

Irbesartan (IS), a selective AT_2-1-R antagonist improved motor functions, reduced infarct size and decreased the number of apoptotic cells particularly in the periinfarct area by attenuated invasion of activated microglia likewise macrophages [82–84].

Losartan (LS), a clinical established selective AT_2-1-R antagonist, did not increase mortality in acute cerebral ischemia [85]. Also, LS (20 µmol/L) abolished ischemic exaggeration of cell injury [26,86]. Expression levels of pro-apoptotic genes were significant reduced by LS treatment [87]. Further LS administration initiates cerebral angiogenic response with a significantly larger vessel surface area, and administration before initiation of cerebral focal ischemia (50 mg/day for 2 weeks) markedly reduces infarct size [88].

3.2. Clinical Studies on Sartans in Ischemic Stroke

The search yielded 19 clinical studies on "Sartans AND ischemic stroke", eligible for systematic review (Table 2). Beneficial aspects of using AT_2-1-R antagonists before the onset of ischemic stroke have already been elucidated in a retrospective analysis of 151 patients [89].

Table 2. Tabular listing of different clinical studies showing various effects of Sartan administration (Abbreviations: Candesartan (CS); hours (h); losartan (LS); milligram (mg); minutes (min); µmol (micromolar); modified ranking Scale (mRS); mol (molar); nmol (nanomolar); telmisartan (TMS); valsartan (VS)).

Drug	Outcome	Beneficial Effect	Special Remarks
CS [90]	Vascular event (vascular death, nonfatal stroke or nonfatal myocardial infarction) over 6 months and mRS	No overall effect on vascular events in ischemic and/or hemorrhagic stroke, adjusted odds ratio for vascular events of patients treated within 6 h reached significance	Administration at least within 30 h of ischemic or hemorrhagic stroke. CS treatment for 7 days, increasing from 4 mg on day 1 to 16 mg on day 3 to 7
CS [91]	Barthel index and level of care assessed after 6 months	No significant effects on Barthel Index or level of care at 6 months	Administration at least within 30 h of ischemic or hemorrhagic stroke. CS treatment for 7 days, increasing from 4 mg on day 1 to 16 mg on day 3 to 7
CS [92]	Vascular death, myocardial infarction, stroke during first 6 months and functional outcome at 6 months	Significant trend towards a better effect of CS in patients with larger infarcts; no differences in treatment effect for composite vascular end point	CS treatment for 7 days, increasing from 4 mg on day 1 to 16 mg on day 3 to 7

Table 2. Cont.

Drug	Outcome	Beneficial Effect	Special Remarks
CS [93]	Vascular death, myocardial infarction, stroke during first 6 months and functional outcome at 6 months	After 6 months the risk of the composite vascular endpoint did not differ between treatment groups	CS treatment for 7 days, increasing from 4 mg on day 1 to 16 mg on day 3 to 7
CS [94]	Safety of modest blood pressure reduction by CS cilexetil in the early treatment of stroke	The cumulative 12 months mortality and the number of vascular events differed significantly in favor of the CS cilexetil group	CS treatment with 4 mg on day 1; dosage increased to 8 mg on day 2 or 16 mg if blood pressure exceeded 160 mmHg systolic or 100 mmHg diastolic
CS [95]	Short-term safety of blood pressure reduction in hypertensive patients with acute ischemic stroke	CS treatment safely reduces blood pressure in hypertensive patients with acute ischemic stroke	4 mg/day for 14 days
CS [96]	Adhesion of neutrophils to human endothelial cells in acute ischemic stroke	CS inhibited the adhesion of neutrophils to vascular endothelium in ischemic stroke patients (not in chronic stroke patients or healthy volunteers)	Incubation with 10^{-9} mol for 30 min
CS [97]	Effect of blood pressure lowering in patients with acute ischemic stroke and carotid artery stenosis (Vascular death, stroke, myocardial infarction, and functional outcome at 6 months)	No evidence that CS effect is qualitatively different in patients with carotid artery stenosis	CS treatment for 7 days, increasing from 4 mg on day 1 to 16 mg on day 3 to 7
VS [98]	Safety of modest blood pressure reduction within 48 h of acute ischemic stroke	After 90 days the mRS as well the rate of major vascular events differed not significantly between both groups	80 mg/day (dose was modified in the subsequent six-days of treatment if the target systolic blood pressure was not achieved)
VS [99]	Effect of vs. on human platelet aggregation	VS exhibited significant inhibition of human platelets and therefore might be able to reduce vascular ischemic events	10 nmol to 100 µmol
TMS [100]	Time to first recurrent stroke	Low glomerular filtration rate (<60 mL/min) is independently associated with a higher risk of recurrent stroke, TMS not able to mitigate this risk	TMS dosage not reported
TMS [101]	Recurrent stroke of any type	Similar rates of recurrent strokes comparing aspirin plus extended-release dipyridamole with clopidogrel and TMS	80 mg/day
TMS [102]	Prevention of cerebral white matter lesions	TMS on top of existing antihypertensive medication did not prevent the progression of white matter lesions	80 mg/day. Analysis limited by the relatively short follow-up
TMS [103]	Functional outcome at 30 days (primary outcome), death, recurrence, and hemodynamic measures up to 90 days (secondary outcomes)	TMS treatment appears to be safe with no excess in adverse events and not associated with a significant effect on functional dependency, death, or stroke recurrence	80 mg/day
TMS [104]	Recurrent stroke	TMS initiated soon after ischemic stroke and continued for 2.5 years did not significantly lower the rate of recurrent stroke, major cardiovascular events, or diabetes	80 mg/day
LS [105]	Global change of cerebral blood flow	LS treatment increases the global cerebral blood flow despite blood pressure lowering	50–100 mg/day for 4 weeks
LS [106]	Effect on stroke in patients with isolated systolic hypertension and left ventricular hypertrophy	Incidence of any stroke (40% risk reduction), fatal stroke (70% risk reduction), and atherothrombotic stroke (45% risk reduction) was significantly lower in the LS treated group compared to atenolol treated patients	Mean LS dose of 79 mg
LS [107]	Effect on global and focal cerebral blood flow in hypertensive patients 2–7 days after stroke	No neurological deterioration in the LS group	25–50 mg/day
LS [108]	Spontaneous platelet aggregation and P-selectin levels (in patients with hypertension and chronic ischemic stroke)	Spontaneous platelet aggregation was not, P-selectin levels significantly reduced after LS treatment. This suggests that standard doses of LS display antiplatelet effect	50 mg/day

CS has been evaluated in the Scandinavian Candesartan Acute Stroke Trial (SCAST). Within 30 h of ischemic or hemorrhagic stroke, 2029 patients either received CS- or placebo-treatment. The modified ranking Scale (mRS) was used for outcome analysis. CS showed no overall effect on vascular events in ischemic and/or hemorrhagic stroke, and the adjusted odds ratio for vascular events of patients treated within 6 h reached significance [90]. At six months, activities of daily living and level of care were assessed. In more than 1800 patients, over 1500 suffered ischemic and almost 250 hemorrhagic strokes. No statistically significant effects of CS on Barthel index or level of care could be identified [91]. Furthermore, the SCAST group evaluated whether the effect of CS treatment varies in subtypes of over 1700 ischemic strokes. Concerning functional outcomes, a trend towards a beneficial effect of CS was observed in patients with larger infarcts (total anterior circulation or partial anterior circulation) than in patients with smaller lacunar infarcts [92]. Further on, over 2000 SCAST patients were randomly allocated to placebo or CS treatment for seven days with increasing doses from 4 mg (starting day 1) to 16 mg (from day 3 to 7). After six months' follow-up, the risk of the composite vascular endpoint did not differ between the placebo and CS treatment group [93]. Also, the Acute Candesartan Cilexetil Therapy in Stroke Survivors study confirmed that administration of CS in the acute phase of stroke in 339 patients confers long-term benefits in patients who sustained acute ischemic stroke [94]. VS has been evaluated in a multicenter trial concerning efficacy and safety of modest blood pressure reduction within 48 h in more than 370 patients with acute ischemic stroke, considering the primary outcome death or dependency. The VS-treated group showed 46 of 187 patients with a 90-day mRS of 3–6, compared with 42 of 185 patients in the control group. The rate of major vascular events did not differ significantly between both groups [98]. TMS has also been evaluated concerning beneficial effects after stroke treatment. A multicenter trial, involving more than 18,500 patients with ischemic stroke, had a follow-up of 2.5 years. The primary outcome parameter was time to first recurrent stroke. Only short-term add-on TMS (80 mg/day) treatment did not mitigate this risk [100,101]. Treatment with TMS (80 mg/day) did not prevent progression of white matter lesions in patients with recent ischemic stroke [102]. Another study group enrolled 20,332 patients and analyzed 1360 patients within 72 h of ischemic stroke onset (TMS vs. placebo) concerning functional outcome after 30 days as primary outcome. Combined death or dependency did not differ between the treatment groups, showing treatment with TMS (80 mg/day) in patients with acute mild ischemic stroke and mildly elevated BP safe with no excess in adverse events [103]. Also, effects of TMS (80 mg/day) initiation early after stroke have been analyzed. From 20,332 patients with recent ischemic stroke, 10,146 patients were randomly assigned in the TMS group and 10,186 in the placebo group; 8.7% in the TMS group and 9.2% in the placebo group suffered from subsequent stroke, showing no significant reduction of recurrent stroke after early initiation [104]. LS has also been analyzed in recent clinical stroke trials. In a double-blinded multi-center trial, 196 hypertensive patients with previous ischemic stroke were randomized to cilnidipine- or LS-treatment (50–100 mg per day for four weeks) once daily for four weeks. Both treatments, however, increased global CBF despite BP lowering [105]. Additionally, the effect of long-term therapy with LS regarding cognitive function in 6206 essential hypertonic patients with additional cerebrovascular risk factors was investigated. The LS-based antihypertensive treatment increased the proportion of patients with normal cognitive function [109]. Also, the Losartan Intervention for Endpoint reduction in hypertension study group reported cardioprotective effects of a LS-based antihypertensive regimen. The incidence of any stroke, fatal stroke, and atherothrombotic stroke was significantly lower in LS-treated compared to the atenolol-treated isolated systolic hypertensive patients [106]. Other groups assessed the effect of LS treatment on mean arterial blood pressure, global, and focal CBF in 24 hypertensive patients without occlusive carotid disease 2–7 days after ischemic stroke and/or transient ischemic attack. LS (25–50 mg per day) was generally well tolerated and none of the patients suffered neurological deterioration. No changes occurred in internal carotid artery flow or cortical as well as hemispheric CBF [107].

3.3. Therapeutic Interventions After aSAH

Poor patients' outcome after aSAH is owed a multifactorial process (early brain injury, DCVS, DCI, cerebral inflammation, cortical spreading depression, loss of pressure dependent cerebral autoregulation) [4,5,7,9,110–113]. DCVS is treated with moderate hypertensive, normovolemic, hemodilution, and in cases of therapy-refractory, DCVS with intra-arterial spasmolysis or balloon dilatation [114,115]. Research to improve poor functional outcome in patients suffering from aSAH and related DCVS is pivotal [1,5,21,116,117]. Multiple preclinical and clinical trials showed the effect of ET-1 in mediating DCVS after aSAH. CONSCIOUS-1, a randomized, double-blind, placebo-controlled study assessed the efficacy of intravenous clazosentan (ET_A-R antagonist) in preventing vasospasm following aSAH. It significantly decreased angiographic DCVS with a trend for reduction in vasospasm-related morbidity/mortality [118]. CONSCIOUS-2 assigned patients with aSAH and clip ligation to clazosentan- or placebo. Thereby, clazosentan showed no significant difference in the mortality and vasospasm-related morbidity [119]. CONSCIOUS-3 assessed whether clazosentan reduced DCVS-related morbidity and mortality after aSAH and endovascular coiling. Pulmonary complications and anemia were more common in patients with clazosentan administration than in the placebo group, and mortality rates after 12 weeks were the same, respectively [120]. The REVERSE-study, infusing clazosentan intravenously in patients developing moderate to severe angiographic vasospasm after aSAH, showed a clear pharmacodynamic dilating effect on DCVS 24 h in most patients suffering aSAH, being able to reverse established angiographic vasospasm [22].

Antihypertensive agents are usually discontinued to maintain a sufficient mean arterial cerebral perfusion pressure considering the prolonged phase of DCVS between days 5 to 14 after the ictus [114]. In contrast, nimodipine, a calcium-channel antagonist, is administered for risk reduction of DCVS, yet rather its neuroprotective effects have been discussed in its beneficial role in aSAH [8,121].

3.4. Effects of Losartan Following aSAH

LS, an already well-established antihypertensive drug in daily clinical practice and well examined in preclinical and clinical settings of ischemic stroke, shows promising results by attenuating cerebral inflammation and restoring cerebral autoregulation [64,105,122–125]. Facing preclinical aSAH research, beneficial effects of Sartans have been shown. Under already physiological conditions, LS diminished cerebral inflammation and associated DCVS [126] as well as ET-1 mediated vasoconstriction. Targeted ET_{B1}- and ET_A-R-antagonism under LS administration revealed a direct modulatory ET_{B1}-R dependent effect via inducing upregulation of the NO-pathway with a significantly increased relaxation accompanied with enhanced sensitivity of the ET_{B1}-R [23]. After induction of aSAH, ET-1-induced vasoconstriction was likewise decreased by LS preincubation, abolished after pretreatment with an ET_{B1}-R antagonist. In precontracted vessels with LS and ET_A-R-antagonism, ET-1 induced a higher vasorelaxation compared to the control group without, clearly demonstrating a modulatory and functional restoring effect of LS on the normally after aSAH impaired ET_{B1}-R function [127].

Beneficial effects of LS on ET-1- and PGF2α-mediated DCVS after aSAH in a rat model have been reported, too [23,127]. An ET-1 mediated vasoconstriction was diminished, and ET_{B1}-R mediated vasorelaxation under selective ET_A-R blockade was restored [126,127]. In addition, PGF2α-elicited vasoconstriction of a basilar artery was markedly diminished [23,126,127]. Interestingly, several work groups could also verify positive vasomodulating effects of LS on the cerebral vessel wall, especially affecting SMCs [128,129]. Furthermore, aneurysm rupture was prevented in mice under LS treatment [129]. As already mentioned, after aSAH, increased synthesis of ET-1 triggers enhanced cerebral vasoconstriction; loss of the ET_{B1}-R mediated vasorelaxation contributes to this effect, too [127]. Furthermore, upregulated AT_2-1-R and PGF2α-synthesis contribute in enhancing and maintaining cerebral vasocontraction [7,130–133]. LS showed promising aspects in preclinical aSAH studies and therefore might have an effect in the treatment of patients with aSAH.

4. Discussions

This systematic review demonstrated Sartan administration after ischemic stroke clearly associated with beneficial effects on preclinical models as well regarding clinical trials. Clear evidence of which doses in preclinical and clinical settings for treatment of ischemic stroke with Sartans exactly might be useful are heterogenous and therefore not consistent yet. In a preclinical setting, Sartans significantly reduced infarct volume and edema, augmented CBF, diminished superoxide production, inflammatory processes, and disruption of the BBB. In clinical studies, clear trends towards a better functional outcome and neurocognitive function after stroke with Sartan use have been reported. Thus, the question arises whether Sartans might provide positive effects on DCVS or DCI after aSAH. In summary, LS provided in a preclinical physiological and pathophysiological setup after aSAH beneficial aspects in reducing ET-1- and PGF2α mediated cerebral vasoconstriction [126,130]. Vasoconstriction was notably reduced and the vasorelaxant properties of the ET_{B1}-R were restored. Furthermore, clear evidence exists, that after aSAH, AT_2-1-R are upregulated in experimental settings [132]. Here, an additive direct antagonism on these receptors could reduce the sensitivity to an AT_2-1-R-mediated vasocontraction to angiotensin II, too [125,134]. LS possesses beneficial aspects on cerebral epileptogenicity, which could be applied to the issue of reducing cortical spreading depression post aSAH [135–138]. Also, it is able to restore post-ischemic cerebral autoregulation after hemorrhagic stroke [134].

Considering these neuroprotective effects of LS, the ethical question arises of whether the philosophy of strictly discontinuing all antihypertensive agents after aSAH (except of new administration of nimodipine), especially of LS, should stay state of the art. Next to beneficial influences on DCVS after aSAH in rats as mentioned above, AT_2-1-R antagonists clearly possess beneficial effects after stroke regarding cerebral inflammation, the areal of infarction, cortical spreading depression, cerebral microcirculation, and maintenance of pressure-dependent cerebral vasoconstriction [23,64,71,105,127,134,139–141]. Appreciating these facts, a systemic LS administration over and above the phase of DCVS, could be a promising approach in preventing these effects; particularly because LS seems to not influence the global CBF in essential hypertonic patients, which can be set equivalent to a needed-hypertonia after aSAH [142]. Here, LS could be an interesting approach, because it increases global CBF despite lowering blood pressure [105], and is therefore capable to reduce DCI [92]. Also, considering the positive vasomodulatory influences of LS, the question arises whether after aSAH this medication should be established as secondary prophylaxis to avoid a de-novo-aneurysm genesis, ergo, if aneurysms under LS are anyway arising [143].

4.1. Translational Aspects

Both abovementioned questions after aSAH are difficult to adapt to the affected patient group, because common sense to date stays in discontinuing all antihypertensive agents after the initial bleeding event. Also, it is vague to postulate that a LS effect persists after discharging this medication on admission over the phase of DCVS for 14 days. Furthermore, the numbers of patients with LS as standard antihypertonic medication receiving follow-up angiographys are too scarce to testify a valid statement concerning case-control studies of aneurysm-growth/-development, as reviewed in our own patient series in 2009–2015. Nevertheless, LS seems to be an underrated neuroprotective drug, reducing cerebral inflammation and epileptogenicity, DCVS, and infarct size after ischemic stroke. These results of preclinical ischemic stroke and aSAH research as well as clinical ischemic stroke research could be applied in a prospective clinical setting of patients suffering aSAH. Also, the question of a de-novo-aneurysm-genesis in further cranial control imaging could be addressed.

4.2. Synopsis and Forecast

LS, a selective AT_2-1-R antagonist, was shown to directly antagonize and ameliorate the impaired ET_{B1}-R vasodilatory function. Given that in most clinical centers, antihypertensive agents are discontinued during the period of DCVS, LS, although an antihypertensive drug, may have a role in preventing delayed DCVS after aneurysm rupture given the effects shown in ischemia. Following aSAH, immediate therapy with LS might antagonize the vasoconstrictive AT_2-1-R without affecting the dilatory AT_2-2-R effect [132,144–151]. Furthermore, AT_2 interestingly increases endothelin production in non-cerebral vessels (an increased ET-1 concentration in rat aortas could be inhibited through LS administration [140]) and thus indirectly enhances ET-1-mediated DCVS [123,152–156]. All these aspects might suggest a crosstalk between both peptidergic systems extra- and intracranially [71,157].

5. Conclusions

There is a promising effect on LS in the treatment of ischemic stroke both in preclinical and clinical studies as well as in preclinical studies on aSAH. LS has shown to reduce ET-1-mediated vasocontraction, cerebral inflammation, and restores vasodilatory function of the ET_{B1}-R [26–28]. Thus, LS may decrease the incidence of symptomatic vasospasm and improve functional outcome in aSAH patients. Large, randomized, double-blinded clinical trials are necessary to determine its benefit in aSAH.

Author Contributions: S.W. and L.A.: Design of the review, collection and analysis of data, drafting the manuscript; B.E.G., S.D.S., H.R.W., S.M., and J.F.: Critical revision of the first draft; All of the authors: Critical revision of the final manuscript. All authors have read and agreed to the published version of the manuscript.

Funding: This research received no external funding.

Conflicts of Interest: The authors declare no conflict of interest.

References

1. Vatter, H.; Konczalla, J.; Weidauer, S.; Preibisch, C.; Zimmermann, M.; Raabe, A.; Seifert, V. Effect of delayed cerebral vasospasm on cerebrovascular endothelin A receptor expression and function. *J. Neurosurg.* **2007**, *107*, 121–127. [CrossRef]
2. Brandt, L.; Ljunggren, B.; Andersson, K.E.; Hindfelt, B.; Uski, T. Prostaglandin metabolism and prostacyclin in cerebral vasospasm. *Gen. Pharmacol.* **1983**, *14*, 141–143. [CrossRef]
3. Egg, D.; Herold, M.; Rumpl, E.; Gunther, R. Prostaglandin F2 alpha levels in human cerebrospinal fluid in normal and pathological conditions. *J. Neurol.* **1980**, *222*, 239–248. [CrossRef] [PubMed]
4. Fujii, M.; Yan, J.; Rolland, W.B.; Soejima, Y.; Caner, B.; Zhang, J.H. Early brain injury, an evolving frontier in subarachnoid hemorrhage research. *Transl. Stroke Res.* **2013**, *4*, 432–446. [CrossRef] [PubMed]
5. Dreier, J.P.; Drenckhahn, C.; Woitzik, J.; Major, S.; Offenhauser, N.; Weber-Carstens, S.; Wolf, S.; Strong, A.J.; Vajkoczy, P.; Hartings, J.A.; et al. Spreading ischemia after aneurysmal subarachnoid hemorrhage. *Acta Neurochir. Suppl.* **2013**, *115*, 125–129. [PubMed]
6. Vergouwen, M.D.; Vermeulen, M.; van Gijn, J.; Rinkel, G.J.; Wijdicks, E.F.; Muizelaar, J.P.; Mendelow, A.D.; Juvela, S.; Yonas, H.; Terbrugge, K.G.; et al. Definition of delayed cerebral ischemia after aneurysmal subarachnoid hemorrhage as an outcome event in clinical trials and observational studies: Proposal of a multidisciplinary research group. *Stroke* **2010**, *41*, 2391–2395. [CrossRef] [PubMed]
7. Budohoski, K.P.; Czosnyka, M.; Smielewski, P.; Kasprowicz, M.; Helmy, A.; Bulters, D.; Pickard, J.D.; Kirkpatrick, P.J. Impairment of cerebral autoregulation predicts delayed cerebral ischemia after subarachnoid hemorrhage: A prospective observational study. *Stroke* **2012**, *43*, 3230–3237. [CrossRef]
8. Bederson, J.B.; Connolly, E.S.; Batjer, H.H., Jr.; Dacey, R.G.; Dion, J.E.; Diringer, M.N.; Duldner, J.E., Jr.; Harbaugh, R.E.; Patel, A.B.; Rosenwasser, R.H.; et al. Guidelines for the management of aneurysmal subarachnoid hemorrhage: A statement for healthcare professionals from a special writing group of the Stroke Council, American Heart Association. *Stroke* **2009**, *40*, 994–1025. [CrossRef]
9. Salom, J.B.; Torregrosa, G.; Alborch, E. Endothelins and the cerebral circulation. *Cerebrovasc. Brain Metab. Rev.* **1995**, *7*, 131–152.
10. Vatter, H.; Zimmermann, M.; Seifert, V.; Schilling, L. Experimental approaches to evaluate endothelin-A receptor antagonists. *Methods Find. Exp. Clin. Pharmacol.* **2004**, *26*, 277–286.
11. Zimmermann, M.; Seifert, V. Endothelin and subarachnoid hemorrhage: An overview. *Neurosurgery* **1998**, *43*, 863–875. [CrossRef] [PubMed]
12. Neuschmelting, V.; Marbacher, S.; Fathi, A.R.; Jakob, S.M.; Fandino, J. Elevated level of endothelin-1 in cerebrospinal fluid and lack of nitric oxide in basilar arterial plasma associated with cerebral vasospasm after subarachnoid haemorrhage in rabbits. *Acta Neurochir.* **2009**, *151*, 795–801. [CrossRef] [PubMed]
13. Josko, J.; Hendryk, S.; Jedrzejowska-Szypulka, H.; Slowinski, J.; Gwozdz, B.; Lange, D.; Harabin-Slowinska, M. Effect of endothelin-1 receptor antagonist BQ-123 on basilar artery diameter after subarachnoid hemorrhage (SAH) in rats. *J. Physiol. Pharmacol.* **2000**, *51*, 241–249. [PubMed]

14. Nishizawa, S.; Chen, D.; Yokoyama, T.; Yokota, N.; Otha, S. Endothelin-1 initiates the development of vasospasm after subarachnoid haemorrhage through protein kinase C activation, but does not contribute to prolonged vasospasm. *Acta Neurochir.* **2000**, *142*, 1409–1415. [CrossRef] [PubMed]
15. Hansen-Schwartz, J.; Hoel, N.L.; Zhou, M.; Xu, C.B.; Svendgaard, N.A.; Edvinsson, L. Subarachnoid hemorrhage enhances endothelin receptor expression and function in rat cerebral arteries. *Neurosurgery* **2003**, *52*, 1188–1194. [PubMed]
16. Lei, Q.; Li, S.; Zheng, R.; Xu, K.; Li, S. Endothelin-1 expression and alterations of cerebral microcirculation after experimental subarachnoid hemorrhage. *Neuroradiology* **2015**, *57*, 63–70. [CrossRef] [PubMed]
17. Josko, J.; Hendryk, S.; Jedrzejowska-Szypulka, H.; Slowinski, J.; Gwozdz, B.; Lange, D.; Snietura, M.; Zwirska-Korczala, K.; Jochem, J. Cerebral angiogenesis after subarachnoid hemorrhage (SAH) and endothelin receptor blockage with BQ-123 antagonist in rats. *J. Physiol. Pharmacol.* **2001**, *52*, 237–248.
18. Xie, A.; Aihara, Y.; Bouryi, V.A.; Nikitina, E.; Jahromi, B.S.; Zhang, Z.D.; Takahashi, M.; Macdonald, R.L. Novel mechanism of endothelin-1-induced vasospasm after subarachnoid hemorrhage. *J. Cereb. Blood Flow Metab.* **2007**, *27*, 1692–1701. [CrossRef]
19. Kim, C.Y.; Paek, S.H.; Seo, B.G.; Kim, J.H.; Han, D.H. Changes in vascular responses of the basilar artery to acetylcholine and endothelin-1 in an experimental rabbit vasospasm model. *Acta Neurochir.* **2003**, *145*, 571–577. [CrossRef]
20. Chow, M.; Dumont, A.S.; Kassell, N.F. Endothelin receptor antagonists and cerebral vasospasm: An update. *Neurosurgery* **2002**, *51*, 1333–1341. [CrossRef]
21. Macdonald, R.L.; Higashida, R.T.; Keller, E.; Mayer, S.A.; Molyneux, A.; Raabe, A.; Vajkoczy, P.; Wanke, I.; Bach, D.; Frey, A.; et al. Randomised trial of clazosentan, an endothelin receptor antagonist, in patients with aneurysmal subarachnoid hemorrhage undergoing surgical clipping (CONSCIOUS-2). *Acta Neurochir. Suppl.* **2013**, *115*, 27–31. [PubMed]
22. Higashida, R.T.; Bruder, N.; Gupta, R.; Guzman, R.; Hmissi, A.; Marr, A.; Mayer, S.A.; Roux, S.; Weidauer, S.; Aldrich, E.F. Reversal of Vasospasm with Clazosentan After Aneurysmal Subarachnoid Hemorrhage: A Pilot Study. *World Neurosurg.* **2019**, *128*, e639–e648. [CrossRef] [PubMed]
23. Konczalla, J.; Wanderer, S.; Mrosek, J.; Schuss, P.; Platz, J.; Güresir, E.; Seifert, V.; Vatter, H. Crosstalk between the angiotensin and endothelin-system in the cerebrovasculature. *Curr. Neurovasc. Res.* **2013**, *10*, 335–345. [CrossRef] [PubMed]
24. Moher, D.; Liberati, A.; Tetzlaff, J.; Altman, D.G.; Group, P. Preferred reporting items for systematic reviews and meta-analyses: The PRISMA statement. *PLoS Med.* **2009**, *6*, e1000097. [CrossRef]
25. Justin, A.; Divakar, S.; Ramanathan, M. Cerebral ischemia induced inflammatory response and altered glutaminergic function mediated through brain AT1 and not AT2 receptor. *Biomed. Pharmacother.* **2018**, *102*, 947–958. [CrossRef]
26. Iwanami, J.; Mogi, M.; Tsukuda, K.; Min, L.J.; Sakata, A.; Jing, F.; Iwai, M.; Horiuchi, M. Low dose of telmisartan prevents ischemic brain damage with peroxisome proliferator-activated receptor-gamma activation in diabetic mice. *J. Hypertens.* **2010**, *28*, 1730–1737. [CrossRef]
27. Kasahara, Y.; Taguchi, A.; Uno, H.; Nakano, A.; Nakagomi, T.; Hirose, H.; Stern, D.M.; Matsuyama, T. Telmisartan suppresses cerebral injury in a murine model of transient focal ischemia. *Brain Res.* **2010**, *1340*, 70–80. [CrossRef]
28. Iwai, M.; Inaba, S.; Tomono, Y.; Kanno, H.; Iwanami, J.; Mogi, M.; Horiuchi, M. Attenuation of focal brain ischemia by telmisartan, an angiotensin II type 1 receptor blocker, in atherosclerotic apolipoprotein E-deficient mice. *Hypertens. Res.* **2008**, *31*, 161–168. [CrossRef]
29. Li, T.; Zhang, Y.; Zhu, B.; Wu, C.; Chen, Y. Telmisartan regulates the development of cerebral ischemia by alleviating endoplasmic reticulum stress. *Pharmazie* **2018**, *73*, 585–588.
30. Gao, Y.; Li, W.; Liu, Y.; Wang, Y.; Zhang, J.; Li, M.; Bu, M. Effect of Telmisartan on Preventing Learning and Memory Deficits Via Peroxisome Proliferator-Activated Receptor-gamma in Vascular Dementia Spontaneously Hypertensive Rats. *J. Stroke Cerebrovasc. Dis.* **2018**, *27*, 277–285. [CrossRef]
31. Ramanathan, M.; Justin, A.; Sudheer, A.; Shanthakumari, S. Comparison of pre- and post-ischemic treatment of telmisartan and nimodipine combination in experimentally induced cerebral ischemia. *Indian J. Exp. Biol.* **2016**, *54*, 560–568.

32. Kono, S.; Kurata, T.; Sato, K.; Omote, Y.; Hishikawa, N.; Yamashita, T.; Deguchi, K.; Abe, K. Neurovascular protection by telmisartan via reducing neuroinflammation in stroke-resistant spontaneously hypertensive rat brain after ischemic stroke. *J. Stroke Cerebrovasc. Dis.* **2015**, *24*, 537–547. [CrossRef] [PubMed]
33. Dupuis, F.; Vincent, J.M.; Liminana, P.; Chillon, J.M.; Capdeville-Atkinson, C.; Atkinson, J. Effects of suboptimal doses of the AT1 receptor blocker, telmisartan, with the angiotensin-converting enzyme inhibitor, ramipril, on cerebral arterioles in spontaneously hypertensive rat. *J. Hypertens.* **2010**, *28*, 1566–1573. [CrossRef] [PubMed]
34. Deguchi, K.; Kurata, T.; Fukui, Y.; Liu, W.; Yun, Z.; Omote, Y.; Sato, K.; Kono, S.; Hishikawa, N.; Yamashita, T.; et al. Long-term amelioration of telmisartan on metabolic syndrome-related molecules in stroke-resistant spontaneously hypertensive rat after transient middle cerebral artery occlusion. *J. Stroke Cerebrovasc. Dis.* **2014**, *23*, 2646–2653. [CrossRef]
35. Thoene-Reineke, C.; Rumschussel, K.; Schmerbach, K.; Krikov, M.; Wengenmayer, C.; Godes, M.; Mueller, S.; Villringer, A.; Steckelings, U.; Namsolleck, P.; et al. Prevention and intervention studies with telmisartan, ramipril and their combination in different rat stroke models. *PLoS ONE* **2011**, *6*, e23646. [CrossRef]
36. Kobayashi, T.; Kawamata, T.; Shibata, N.; Okada, Y.; Kobayashi, M.; Hori, T. Angiotensin II type 1 receptor blocker telmisartan reduces cerebral infarct volume and peri-infarct cytosolic phospholipase A(2) level in experimental stroke. *J. Neurotrauma.* **2009**, *26*, 2355–2364. [CrossRef]
37. Jung, K.H.; Chu, K.; Lee, S.T.; Kim, S.J.; Song, E.C.; Kim, E.H.; Park, D.K.; Sinn, D.I.; Kim, J.M.; Kim, M. Blockade of AT1 receptor reduces apoptosis, inflammation, and oxidative stress in normotensive rats with intracerebral hemorrhage. *J. Pharmacol. Exp. Ther.* **2007**, *322*, 1051–1058. [CrossRef]
38. Fukui, Y.; Yamashita, T.; Kurata, T.; Sato, K.; Lukic, V.; Hishikawa, N.; Deguchi, K.; Abe, K. Protective effect of telmisartan against progressive oxidative brain damage and synuclein phosphorylation in stroke-resistant spontaneously hypertensive rats. *J. Stroke Cerebrovasc. Dis.* **2014**, *23*, 1545–1553. [CrossRef]
39. Hamai, M.; Iwai, M.; Ide, A.; Tomochika, H.; Tomono, Y.; Mogi, M.; Horiuchi, M. Comparison of inhibitory action of candesartan and enalapril on brain ischemia through inhibition of oxidative stress. *Neuropharmacology* **2006**, *51*, 822–828. [CrossRef]
40. Awad, A.S. Effect of combined treatment with curcumin and candesartan on ischemic brain damage in mice. *J. Stroke Cerebrovasc. Dis.* **2011**, *20*, 541–548. [CrossRef]
41. Soliman, S.; Ishrat, T.; Fouda, A.Y.; Patel, A.; Pillai, B.; Fagan, S.C. Sequential Therapy with Minocycline and Candesartan Improves Long-Term Recovery After Experimental Stroke. *Transl. Stroke Res.* **2015**, *6*, 309–322. [CrossRef] [PubMed]
42. Ishrat, T.; Soliman, S.; Eldahshan, W.; Pillai, B.; Ergul, A.; Fagan, S.C. Silencing VEGF-B Diminishes the Neuroprotective Effect of Candesartan Treatment After Experimental Focal Cerebral Ischemia. *Neurochem. Res.* **2018**, *43*, 1869–1878. [CrossRef] [PubMed]
43. Culman, J.; Jacob, T.; Schuster, S.O.; Brolund-Spaether, K.; Brolund, L.; Cascorbi, I.; Zhao, Y.; Gohlke, P. Neuroprotective effects of AT1 receptor antagonists after experimental ischemic stroke: What is important? *Naunyn. Schmiedebergs Arch. Pharmacol.* **2017**, *390*, 949–959. [CrossRef] [PubMed]
44. Alhusban, A.; Kozak, A.; Pillai, B.; Ahmed, H.; Sayed, M.A.; Johnson, M.H.; Ishrat, T.; Ergul, A.; Fagan, S.C. Mechanisms of acute neurovascular protection with AT1 blockade after stroke: Effect of prestroke hypertension. *PLoS ONE* **2017**, *12*, e0178867. [CrossRef]
45. Fouda, A.Y.; Alhusban, A.; Ishrat, T.; Pillai, B.; Eldahshan, W.; Waller, J.L.; Ergul, A.; Fagan, S.C. Brain-Derived Neurotrophic Factor Knockdown Blocks the Angiogenic and Protective Effects of Angiotensin Modulation After Experimental Stroke. *Mol. Neurobiol.* **2017**, *54*, 661–670. [CrossRef]
46. Soliman, S.; Ishrat, T.; Pillai, A.; Somanath, P.R.; Ergul, A.; El-Remessy, A.B.; Fagan, S.C. Candesartan induces a prolonged proangiogenic effect and augments endothelium-mediated neuroprotection after oxygen and glucose deprivation: Role of vascular endothelial growth factors A and B. *J. Pharmacol. Exp. Ther.* **2014**, *349*, 444–457. [CrossRef]
47. Alhusban, A.; Kozak, A.; Ergul, A.; Fagan, S.C. AT1 receptor antagonism is proangiogenic in the brain: BDNF a novel mediator. *J. Pharmacol. Exp. Ther.* **2013**, *344*, 348–359. [CrossRef]
48. So, G.; Nakagawa, S.; Morofuji, Y.; Hiu, T.; Hayashi, K.; Tanaka, K.; Suyama, K.; Deli, M.A.; Nagata, I.; Matsuo, T.; et al. Candesartan improves ischemia-induced impairment of the blood-brain barrier in vitro. *Cell Mol. Neurobiol.* **2015**, *35*, 563–572. [CrossRef]

49. Panahpour, H.; Nekooeian, A.A.; Dehghani, G.A. Candesartan attenuates ischemic brain edema and protects the blood-brain barrier integrity from ischemia/reperfusion injury in rats. *Iran. Biomed. J.* **2014**, *18*, 232–238.
50. Ishrat, T.; Pillai, B.; Soliman, S.; Fouda, A.Y.; Kozak, A.; Johnson, M.H.; Ergul, A.; Fagan, S.C. Low-dose candesartan enhances molecular mediators of neuroplasticity and subsequent functional recovery after ischemic stroke in rats. *Mol. Neurobiol.* **2015**, *51*, 1542–1553. [CrossRef]
51. Guan, W.; Kozak, A.; Fagan, S.C. Drug repurposing for vascular protection after acute ischemic stroke. *Acta Neurochir. Suppl.* **2011**, *111*, 295–298. [PubMed]
52. Schmerbach, K.; Pfab, T.; Zhao, Y.; Culman, J.; Mueller, S.; Villringer, A.; Muller, D.N.; Hocher, B.; Unger, T.; Thoene-Reineke, C. Effects of aliskiren on stroke in rats expressing human renin and angiotensinogen genes. *PLoS ONE* **2010**, *5*, e15052. [CrossRef] [PubMed]
53. Omura-Matsuoka, E.; Yagita, Y.; Sasaki, T.; Terasaki, Y.; Oyama, N.; Sugiyama, Y.; Okazaki, S.; Ssakoda, S.; Kitagawa, K. Postischemic administration of angiotensin II type 1 receptor blocker reduces cerebral infarction size in hypertensive rats. *Hypertens. Res.* **2009**, *32*, 548–553. [CrossRef]
54. Kozak, W.; Kozak, A.; Johnson, M.H.; Elewa, H.F.; Fagan, S.C. Vascular protection with candesartan after experimental acute stroke in hypertensive rats: A dose-response study. *J. Pharmacol. Exp. Ther.* **2008**, *326*, 773–782. [CrossRef] [PubMed]
55. Krikov, M.; Thone-Reineke, C.; Muller, S.; Villringer, A.; Unger, T. Candesartan but not ramipril pretreatment improves outcome after stroke and stimulates neurotrophin BNDF/TrkB system in rats. *J. Hypertens.* **2008**, *26*, 544–552. [CrossRef] [PubMed]
56. Fagan, S.C.; Kozak, A.; Hill, W.D.; Pollock, D.M.; Xu, L.; Johnson, M.H.; Ergul, A.; Hess, D.C. Hypertension after experimental cerebral ischemia: Candesartan provides neurovascular protection. *J. Hypertens.* **2006**, *24*, 535–539. [CrossRef] [PubMed]
57. Lu, Q.; Zhu, Y.Z.; Wong, P.T. Neuroprotective effects of candesartan against cerebral ischemia in spontaneously hypertensive rats. *Neuroreport* **2005**, *16*, 1963–1967. [CrossRef]
58. Kusaka, I.; Kusaka, G.; Zhou, C.; Ishikawa, M.; Nanda, A.; Granger, D.N.; Zhang, J.H.; Tang, J. Role of AT1 receptors and NAD(P)H oxidase in diabetes-aggravated ischemic brain injury. *Am. J. Physiol. Heart Circ. Physiol.* **2004**, *286*, H2442–H2451. [CrossRef]
59. Groth, W.; Blume, A.; Gohlke, P.; Unger, T.; Culman, J. Chronic pretreatment with candesartan improves recovery from focal cerebral ischaemia in rats. *J. Hypertens.* **2003**, *21*, 2175–2182. [CrossRef]
60. Nishimura, Y.; Ito, T.; Saavedra, J.M. Angiotensin II AT(1) blockade normalizes cerebrovascular autoregulation and reduces cerebral ischemia in spontaneously hypertensive rats. *Stroke* **2000**, *31*, 2478–2486. [CrossRef]
61. Gaur, V.; Kumar, A. Neuroprotective potentials of candesartan, atorvastatin and their combination against stroke induced motor dysfunction. *Inflammopharmacology* **2011**, *19*, 205–214. [CrossRef] [PubMed]
62. Engelhorn, T.; Doerfler, A.; Heusch, G.; Schulz, R. Reduction of cerebral infarct size by the AT1-receptor blocker candesartan, the HMG-CoA reductase inhibitor rosuvastatin and their combination. An experimental study in rats. *Neurosci. Lett.* **2006**, *406*, 92–96. [CrossRef] [PubMed]
63. Mecca, A.P.; O'Connor, T.E.; Katovich, M.J.; Sumners, C. Candesartan pretreatment is cerebroprotective in a rat model of endothelin-1-induced middle cerebral artery occlusion. *Exp. Physiol.* **2009**, *94*, 937–946. [CrossRef] [PubMed]
64. Schmerbach, K.; Schefe, J.H.; Krikov, M.; Müller, S.; Villringer, A.; Kintscher, U.; Unger, T.; Thoene-Reineke, C. Comparison between single and combined treatment with candesartan and pioglitazone following transient focal ischemia in rat brain. *Brain Res.* **2008**, *1208*, 225–233. [CrossRef] [PubMed]
65. Zhou, J.; Pavel, J.; Macova, M.; Yu, Z.X.; Imboden, H.; Ge, L.; Nishioku, T.; Dou, J.; Delgiacco, E.; Saavedra, J.M. AT1 receptor blockade regulates the local angiotensin II system in cerebral microvessels from spontaneously hypertensive rats. *Stroke* **2006**, *37*, 1271–1276. [CrossRef] [PubMed]
66. Kozak, A.; Ergul, A.; El-Remessy, A.B.; Johnson, M.H.; Machado, L.S.; Elewa, H.F.; Abdelsaid, M.; Wiley, D.C.; Fagan, S.C. Candesartan augments ischemia-induced proangiogenic state and results in sustained improvement after stroke. *Stroke* **2009**, *40*, 1870–1876. [CrossRef] [PubMed]
67. Faure, S.; Bureau, A.; Oudart, N.; Javellaud, J.; Fournier, A.; Achard, J.M. Protective effect of candesartan in experimental ischemic stroke in the rat mediated by AT2 and AT4 receptors. *J. Hypertens.* **2008**, *26*, 2008–2015. [CrossRef]

68. Stenman, E.; Jamali, R.; Henriksson, M.; Maddahi, A.; Edvinsson, L. Cooperative effect of angiotensin AT(1) and endothelin ET(A) receptor antagonism limits the brain damage after ischemic stroke in rat. *Eur. J. Pharmacol.* **2007**, *570*, 142–148. [CrossRef]
69. Stenman, E.; Edvinsson, L. Cerebral ischemia enhances vascular angiotensin AT1 receptor-mediated contraction in rats. *Stroke* **2004**, *35*, 970–974. [CrossRef]
70. Brdon, J.; Kaiser, S.; Hagemann, F.; Zhao, Y.; Culman, J.; Gohlke, P. Comparison between early and delayed systemic treatment with candesartan of rats after ischaemic stroke. *J. Hypertens.* **2007**, *25*, 187–196. [CrossRef] [PubMed]
71. Engelhorn, T.; Goerike, S.; Doerfler, A.; Okorn, C.; Forsting, M.; Heusch, G.; Schulz, R. The angiotensin II type 1-receptor blocker candesartan increases cerebral blood flow, reduces infarct size, and improves neurologic outcome after transient cerebral ischemia in rats. *J. Cereb. Blood Flow Metab.* **2004**, *24*, 467–474. [CrossRef] [PubMed]
72. Yamakawa, H.; Jezova, M.; Ando, H.; Saavedra, J.M. Normalization of endothelial and inducible nitric oxide synthase expression in brain microvessels of spontaneously hypertensive rats by angiotensin II AT1 receptor inhibition. *J. Cereb. Blood Flow Metab.* **2003**, *23*, 371–380. [CrossRef] [PubMed]
73. Nakagawa, T.; Hasegawa, Y.; Uekawa, K.; Senju, S.; Nakagata, N.; Matsui, K.; Kim-Mitsuyama, S. Transient Mild Cerebral Ischemia Significantly Deteriorated Cognitive Impairment in a Mouse Model of Alzheimer's Disease via Angiotensin AT1 Receptor. *Am. J. Hypertens.* **2017**, *30*, 141–150. [CrossRef] [PubMed]
74. Faure, S.; Oudart, N.; Javellaud, J.; Fournier, A.; Warnock, D.G.; Achard, J.M. Synergistic protective effects of erythropoietin and olmesartan on ischemic stroke survival and post-stroke memory dysfunctions in the gerbil. *J. Hypertens.* **2006**, *24*, 2255–2261. [CrossRef] [PubMed]
75. Gutierrez-Fernandez, M.; Fuentes, B.; Rodriguez-Frutos, B.; Ramos-Cejudo, J.; Otero-Ortega, L.; Diez-Tejedor, E. Different protective and reparative effects of olmesartan in stroke according to time of administration and withdrawal. *J. Neurosci. Res.* **2015**, *93*, 806–814. [CrossRef] [PubMed]
76. Oyama, N.; Yagita, Y.; Sasaki, T.; Omura-Matsuoka, E.; Terasaki, Y.; Sugiyama, Y.; Sakoda, S.; Kitagawa, K. An angiotensin II type 1 receptor blocker can preserve endothelial function and attenuate brain ischemic damage in spontaneously hypertensive rats. *J. Neurosci. Res.* **2010**, *88*, 2889–2898. [CrossRef]
77. Hosomi, N.; Nishiyama, A.; Ban, C.R.; Naya, T.; Takahashi, T.; Kohno, M.; Koziol, J.A. Angiotensin type 1 receptor blockage improves ischemic injury following transient focal cerebral ischemia. *Neuroscience* **2005**, *134*, 225–231. [CrossRef]
78. Li, J.M.; Mogi, M.; Iwanami, J.; Min, L.J.; Tsukuda, K.; Sakata, A.; Fujita, T.; Iwai, M.; Horiuchi, M. Temporary pretreatment with the angiotensin II type 1 receptor blocker, valsartan, prevents ischemic brain damage through an increase in capillary density. *Stroke* **2008**, *39*, 2029–2036. [CrossRef]
79. Miyamoto, N.; Zhang, N.; Tanaka, R.; Liu, M.; Hattori, N.; Urabe, T. Neuroprotective role of angiotensin II type 2 receptor after transient focal ischemia in mice brain. *Neurosci. Res.* **2008**, *61*, 249–256. [CrossRef]
80. Iwai, M.; Liu, H.W.; Chen, R.; Ide, A.; Okamoto, S.; Hata, R.; Sakanaka, M.; Shiuchi, T.; Horiuchi, M. Possible inhibition of focal cerebral ischemia by angiotensin II type 2 receptor stimulation. *Circulation* **2004**, *110*, 843–848. [CrossRef]
81. Dong, Y.F.; Kataoka, K.; Tokutomi, Y.; Nako, H.; Nakamura, T.; Toyama, K.; Sueta, D.; Koibuchi, N.; Yamamoto, E.; Ogawa, H.; et al. Beneficial effects of combination of valsartan and amlodipine on salt-induced brain injury in hypertensive rats. *J. Pharmacol. Exp. Ther.* **2011**, *339*, 358–366. [CrossRef] [PubMed]
82. Lou, M.; Blume, A.; Zhao, Y.; Gohlke, P.; Deuschl, G.; Herdegen, T.; Culman, J. Sustained blockade of brain AT1 receptors before and after focal cerebral ischemia alleviates neurologic deficits and reduces neuronal injury, apoptosis, and inflammatory responses in the rat. *J. Cereb. Blood Flow Metab.* **2004**, *24*, 536–547. [CrossRef] [PubMed]
83. Dai, W.J.; Funk, A.; Herdegen, T.; Unger, T.; Culman, J. Blockade of central angiotensin AT(1) receptors improves neurological outcome and reduces expression of AP-1 transcription factors after focal brain ischemia in rats. *Stroke* **1999**, *30*, 2391–2398. [CrossRef]
84. Tsukuda, K.; Mogi, M.; Iwanami, J.; Min, L.J.; Jing, F.; Oshima, K.; Horiuchi, M. Irbesartan attenuates ischemic brain damage by inhibition of MCP-1/CCR2 signaling pathway beyond AT(1) receptor blockade. *Biochem. Biophys. Res. Commun.* **2011**, *409*, 275–279. [CrossRef]

85. Dalmay, F.; Mazouz, H.; Allard, J.; Pesteil, F.; Achard, J.M.; Fournier, A. Non-AT(1)-receptor-mediated protective effect of angiotensin against acute ischaemic stroke in the gerbil. *J. Renin Angiotensin Aldosterone Syst.* **2001**, *2*, 103–106. [CrossRef]
86. Chen, S.; Li, G.; Zhang, W.; Sigmund, C.D.; Olson, J.E.; Chen, Y. Ischemia-induced brain damage is enhanced in human renin and angiotensinogen double-transgenic mice. *Am. J. Physiol. Regul. Integr. Comp. Physiol.* **2009**, *297*, R1526–R1531. [CrossRef]
87. Loh, K.P.; Low, L.S.; Wong, W.H.; Zhou, S.; Huang, S.H.; De Silva, R.; Duan, W.; Chou, W.H.; Zhu, Y.Z. A comparison study of cerebral protection using Ginkgo biloba extract and Losartan on stroked rats. *Neurosci. Lett.* **2006**, *398*, 28–33. [CrossRef]
88. Forder, J.P.; Munzenmaier, D.H.; Greene, A.S. Angiogenic protection from focal ischemia with angiotensin II type 1 receptor blockade in the rat. *Am. J. Physiol. Heart Circ. Physiol.* **2005**, *288*, H1989–H1996. [CrossRef]
89. Miyamoto, N.; Tanaka, Y.; Ueno, Y.; Tanaka, R.; Hattori, N.; Urabe, T. Benefits of prestroke use of angiotensin type 1 receptor blockers on ischemic stroke severity. *J. Stroke Cerebrovasc. Dis.* **2012**, *21*, 363–368. [CrossRef]
90. Jusufovic, M.; Sandset, E.C.; Bath, P.M.; Berge, E.; Scandinavian Candesartan Acute Stroke Trial Study Group. Early blood pressure lowering treatment in acute stroke. Ordinal analysis of vascular events in the Scandinavian Candesartan Acute Stroke Trial (SCAST). *J. Hypertens.* **2016**, *34*, 1594–1598. [CrossRef]
91. Hornslien, A.G.; Sandset, E.C.; Wyller, T.B.; Berge, E.; Scandinavian Candesartan Acute Stroke Trial Study Group. Effects of candesartan in acute stroke on activities of daily living and level of care at 6 months. *J. Hypertens.* **2015**, *33*, 1487–1491. [CrossRef] [PubMed]
92. Sandset, E.C.; Jusufovic, M.; Sandset, P.M.; Bath, P.M.; Berge, E.; Group, S.S. Effects of blood pressure-lowering treatment in different subtypes of acute ischemic stroke. *Stroke* **2015**, *46*, 877–879. [CrossRef] [PubMed]
93. Sandset, E.C.; Bath, P.M.; Boysen, G.; Jatuzis, D.; Korv, J.; Lüders, S.; Murray, G.D.; Richter, P.S.; Roine, R.O.; Terent, A.; et al. The angiotensin-receptor blocker candesartan for treatment of acute stroke (SCAST): A randomised, placebo-controlled, double-blind trial. *Lancet* **2011**, *377*, 741–750. [CrossRef]
94. Schrader, J.; Luders, S.; Kulschewski, A.; Berger, J.; Zidek, W.; Treib, J.; Einhäupl, K.; Diener, H.C.; Dominiak, P.; Acute Candesartan Cilexetil Therapy in Stroke Survivors Study Group. The ACCESS Study: Evaluation of Acute Candesartan Cilexetil Therapy in Stroke Survivors. *Stroke* **2003**, *34*, 1699–1703. [CrossRef]
95. Nakamura, T.; Tsutsumi, Y.; Shimizu, Y.; Uchiyama, S. Renin-angiotensin system blockade safely reduces blood pressure in patients with minor ischemic stroke during the acute phase. *J. Stroke Cerebrovasc. Dis.* **2010**, *19*, 435–440. [CrossRef]
96. Hallevi, H.; Hazan-Halevy, I.; Paran, E. Modification of neutrophil adhesion to human endothelial cell line in acute ischemic stroke by dipyridamole and candesartan. *Eur. J. Neurol.* **2007**, *14*, 1002–1007. [CrossRef]
97. Jusufovic, M.; Sandset, E.C.; Bath, P.M.; Karlson, B.W.; Berge, E.; Scandinavian Candesartan Acute Stroke Trial Study Group. Effects of blood pressure lowering in patients with acute ischemic stroke and carotid artery stenosis. *Int. J. Stroke* **2015**, *10*, 354–359. [CrossRef]
98. Oh, M.S.; Yu, K.H.; Hong, K.S.; Kang, D.W.; Park, J.M.; Bae, H.J.; Koo, J.; Lee, J.; Lee, B.C.; Valsartan Efficacy oN modesT blood pressUre Reduction in acute ischemic stroke (VENTURE) study group. Modest blood pressure reduction with valsartan in acute ischemic stroke: A prospective, randomized, open-label, blinded-end-point trial. *Int. J. Stroke* **2015**, *10*, 745–751. [CrossRef]
99. Serebruany, V.L.; Malinin, A.I.; Lowry, D.R.; Sane, D.C.; Webb, R.L.; Gottlieb, S.O.; O'Connor, C.M.; Hennekens, C.H. Effects of valsartan and valeryl 4-hydroxy valsartan on human platelets: A possible additional mechanism for clinical benefits. *J. Cardiovasc. Pharmacol.* **2004**, *43*, 677–684. [CrossRef]
100. Ovbiagele, B.; Bath, P.M.; Cotton, D.; Sha, N.; Diener, H.C.; Investigators, P.R. Low glomerular filtration rate, recurrent stroke risk, and effect of renin-angiotensin system modulation. *Stroke* **2013**, *44*, 3223–3225. [CrossRef]
101. Wadiwala, M.F.; Kamal, A.K. What is better antiplatelet agent to prevent recurrent stroke? *J. Pak. Med. Assoc.* **2012**, *62*, 976–977. [PubMed]
102. Weber, R.; Weimar, C.; Blatchford, J.; Hermansson, K.; Wanke, I.; Möller-Hartmann, C.; Gizweksi, E.R.; Forsting, M.; Demchuck, A.M.; Sacco, R.L.; et al. Telmisartan on top of antihypertensive treatment does not prevent progression of cerebral white matter lesions in the prevention regimen for effectively avoiding second strokes (PRoFESS) MRI substudy. *Stroke* **2012**, *43*, 2336–2342. [CrossRef] [PubMed]

103. Bath, P.M.; Martin, R.H.; Palesch, Y.; Cotton, D.; Yusuf, S.; Saccor, R.; Diener, H.C.; Toni, D.; Estol, C.; Roberts, R.; et al. Effect of telmisartan on functional outcome, recurrence, and blood pressure in patients with acute mild ischemic stroke: A PRoFESS subgroup analysis. *Stroke* **2009**, *40*, 3541–3546. [CrossRef] [PubMed]
104. Yusuf, S.; Diener, H.C.; Sacco, R.L.; Cotton, D.; Ounpuu, S.; Lawton, W.A.; Palesch, Y.; Martin, R.H.; Albers, G.W.; Bath, P.; et al. Telmisartan to prevent recurrent stroke and cardiovascular events. *N. Engl. J. Med.* **2008**, *359*, 1225–1237. [CrossRef]
105. Hong, K.S.; Kang, D.W.; Bae, H.J.; Kim, Y.K.; Han, M.K.; Park, J.M.; Rha, J.H.; Lee, Y.S.; Koo, J.S.; Cho, Y.J.; et al. Effect of cilnidipine vs. losartan on cerebral blood flow in hypertensive patients with a history of ischemic stroke: A randomized controlled trial. *Acta Neurol. Scand.* **2010**, *121*, 51–57. [CrossRef]
106. Kjeldsen, S.E.; Lyle, P.A.; Kizer, J.R.; Dahlhöf, B.; Devereux, R.B.; Julius, S.; Beevers, G.; de Faire, U.; Fyhrquist, F.; Ibsen, H.; et al. The effects of losartan compared to atenolol on stroke in patients with isolated systolic hypertension and left ventricular hypertrophy. The LIFE study. *J. Clin. Hypertens.* **2005**, *7*, 152–158. [CrossRef]
107. Nazir, F.S.; Overell, J.R.; Bolster, A.; Hilditch, T.E.; Reid, J.L.; Lees, K.R. The effect of losartan on global and focal cerebral perfusion and on renal function in hypertensives in mild early ischaemic stroke. *J. Hypertens.* **2004**, *22*, 989–995. [CrossRef]
108. Yamada, K.; Hirayama, T.; Hasegawa, Y. Antiplatelet effect of losartan and telmisartan in patients with ischemic stroke. *J. Stroke Cerebrovasc. Dis.* **2007**, *16*, 225–231. [CrossRef]
109. Van Ginneken, V.; Engel, P.; Fiebach, J.B.; Audebert, H.J.; Nolte, C.H.; Rocco, A. Prior antiplatelet therapy is not associated with larger hematoma volume or hematoma growth in intracerebral hemorrhage. *Neurol. Sci.* **2018**, *39*, 745–748. [CrossRef]
110. Vatter, H.; Konczalla, J.; Seifert, V. Endothelin related pathophysiology in cerebral vasospasm: What happens to the cerebral vessels? *Acta Neurochir. Suppl.* **2011**, *110*, 177–180.
111. Provencio, J.J. Inflammation in subarachnoid hemorrhage and delayed deterioration associated with vasospasm: A review. *Acta Neurochir. Suppl.* **2013**, *115*, 233–238. [PubMed]
112. Larysz-Brysz, M.; Lewin-Kowalik, J.; Czuba, Z.; Kotulska, K.; Olakowska, E.; Marcol, W.; Liskiewicz, A.; Jedrzejowska-Szypulka, H. Interleukin-1beta increases release of endothelin-1 and tumor necrosis factor as well as reactive oxygen species by peripheral leukocytes during experimental subarachnoid hemorrhage. *Curr. Neurovasc. Res.* **2012**, *9*, 159–166. [CrossRef] [PubMed]
113. Paczkowska, E.; Golab-Janowska, M.; Bajer-Czajkowska, A.; Machalinska, A.; Ustianowski, P.; Rybicka, M.; Klos, P.; Dziedziejko, V.; Safranow, K.; Nowacki, P. Increased circulating endothelial progenitor cells in patients with haemorrhagic and ischaemic stroke: The role of endothelin-1. *J. Neurol. Sci.* **2013**, *325*, 90–99. [CrossRef] [PubMed]
114. Andereggen, L.; Beck, J.; Z'Graggen, W.J.; Schroth, G.; Andres, R.H.; Murek, M.; Haenggi, M.; Reinert, M.; Raabe, A.; Gralla, J. Feasibility and Safety of Repeat Instant Endovascular Interventions in Patients with Refractory Cerebral Vasospasms. *AJNR Am. J. Neuroradiol.* **2017**, *38*, 561–567. [CrossRef]
115. Hosmann, A.; Rauscher, S.; Wang, W.T.; Dodier, P.; Bavinzski, G.; Knosp, E.; Gruber, A. Intra-Arterial Papaverine-Hydrochloride and Transluminal Balloon Angioplasty for Neurointerventional Management of Delayed-Onset Post-Aneurysmal Subarachnoid Hemorrhage Vasospasm. *World Neurosurg.* **2018**, *119*, e301–e312. [CrossRef]
116. Macdonald, R.L.; Higashida, R.T.; Keller, E.; Mayer, S.A.; Molyneux, A.; Raabe, A.; Vajkoczy, P.; Wanke, I.; Frey, A.; Marr, A.; et al. Preventing vasospasm improves outcome after aneurysmal subarachnoid hemorrhage: Rationale and design of CONSCIOUS-2 and CONSCIOUS-3 trials. *Neurocrit. Care* **2010**, *13*, 416–424. [CrossRef]
117. Raabe, A.; Beck, J.; Keller, M.; Vatter, H.; Zimmermann, M.; Seifert, V. Relative importance of hypertension compared with hypervolemia for increasing cerebral oxygenation in patients with cerebral vasospasm after subarachnoid hemorrhage. *J. Neurosurg.* **2005**, *103*, 974–981. [CrossRef]
118. Macdonald, R.L.; Kassell, N.F.; Mayer, S.; Ruefenacht, D.; Schmiedek, P.; Weidauer, S.; Frey, A.; Roux, S.; Pasqualin, A.; CONSCIOUS-1 Investigators. Clazosentan to overcome neurological ischemia and infarction occurring after subarachnoid hemorrhage (CONSCIOUS-1): Randomized, double-blind, placebo-controlled phase 2 dose-finding trial. *Stroke* **2008**, *39*, 3015–3021. [CrossRef]

119. Macdonald, R.L.; Higashida, R.T.; Keller, E.; Mayer, S.A.; Molyneux, A.; Raabe, A.; Vajkoczy, P.; Wanke, I.; Bach, D.; Frey, A.; et al. Clazosentan, an endothelin receptor antagonist, in patients with aneurysmal subarachnoid haemorrhage undergoing surgical clipping: A randomised, double-blind, placebo-controlled phase 3 trial (CONSCIOUS-2). *Lancet Neurol.* **2011**, *10*, 618–625. [CrossRef]
120. Macdonald, R.L.; Higashida, R.T.; Keller, E.; Mayer, S.A.; Molyneux, A.; Raabe, A.; Vajkoczy, P.; Wanke, I.; Bach, D.; Frey, A.; et al. Randomized trial of clazosentan in patients with aneurysmal subarachnoid hemorrhage undergoing endovascular coiling. *Stroke* **2012**, *43*, 1463–1469. [CrossRef]
121. Loch Macdonald, R. Management of cerebral vasospasm. *Neurosurg. Rev.* **2006**, *29*, 179–193. [CrossRef] [PubMed]
122. Rodrigues, S.F.; Granger, D.N. Cerebral microvascular inflammation in DOCA salt-induced hypertension: Role of angiotensin II and mitochondrial superoxide. *J. Cereb. Blood Flow Metab.* **2012**, *32*, 368–375. [CrossRef] [PubMed]
123. Zhang, R.; Witkowski, S.; Fu, Q.; Claassen, J.A.; Levine, B.D. Cerebral hemodynamics after short- and long-term reduction in blood pressure in mild and moderate hypertension. *Hypertension* **2007**, *49*, 1149–1155. [CrossRef] [PubMed]
124. Andereggen, L.; Neuschmelting, V.; von Gunten, M.; Widmer, H.R.; Fandino, J.; Marbacher, S. The role of microclot formation in an acute subarachnoid hemorrhage model in the rabbit. *Biomed. Res. Int.* **2014**, *2014*, 161702. [CrossRef]
125. Bar-Klein, G.; Cacheaux, L.P.; Kamintsky, L.; Prager, O.; Weissberg, I.; Schoknecht, K.; Cheng, P.; Kim, S.Y.; Wood, L.; Heinemann, U.; et al. Losartan prevents acquired epilepsy via TGF-beta signaling suppression. *Ann. Neurol.* **2014**, *75*, 864–875. [CrossRef]
126. Wanderer, S.; Mrosek, J.; Gessler, F.; Seifert, V.; Konczalla, J. Vasomodulatory effects of the angiotensin II type 1 receptor antagonist losartan on experimentally induced cerebral vasospasm after subarachnoid haemorrhage. *Acta Neurochir.* **2018**, *160*, 277–284. [CrossRef]
127. Wanderer, S.; Mrosek, J.; Vatter, H.; Seifert, V.; Konczalla, J. Crosstalk between the angiotensin and endothelin system in the cerebrovasculature after experimental induced subarachnoid hemorrhage. *Neurosurg. Rev.* **2018**, *41*, 539–548. [CrossRef]
128. Gomez-Garre, D.; Martin-Ventura, J.L.; Granados, R.; Sancho, T.; Torres, R.; Ruano, M.; Garcia-Puig, J.; Egido, J. Losartan improves resistance artery lesions and prevents CTGF and TGF-beta production in mild hypertensive patients. *Kidney Int.* **2006**, *69*, 1237–1244. [CrossRef]
129. Tada, Y.; Wada, K.; Shimada, K.; Makino, H.; Liang, E.I.; Murakami, S.; Kudo, M.; Kitazato, K.T.; Nagahiro, S.; Hashimoto, T. Roles of hypertension in the rupture of intracranial aneurysms. *Stroke* **2014**, *45*, 579–586. [CrossRef]
130. Asaeda, M.; Sakamoto, M.; Kurosaki, M.; Tabuchi, S.; Kamitani, H.; Yokota, M.; Watanabe, T. A non-enzymatic derived arachidonyl peroxide, 8-iso-prostaglandin F2 alpha, in cerebrospinal fluid of patients with aneurysmal subarachnoid hemorrhage participates in the pathogenesis of delayed cerebral vasospasm. *Neurosci. Lett.* **2005**, *373*, 222–225. [CrossRef]
131. Konczalla, J.; Vatter, H.; Weidauer, S.; Raabe, A.; Seifert, V. Alteration of the cerebrovascular function of endothelin B receptor after subarachnoidal hemorrhage in the rat. *Exp. Biol. Med.* **2006**, *231*, 1064–1068.
132. Ansar, S.; Vikman, P.; Nielsen, M.; Edvinsson, L. Cerebrovascular ETB, 5-HT1B, and AT1 receptor upregulation correlates with reduction in regional CBF after subarachnoid hemorrhage. *Am. J. Physiol. Heart Circ. Physiol.* **2007**, *293*, H3750–H3758. [CrossRef] [PubMed]
133. Sakamoto, M.; Takaki, E.; Yamashita, K.; Watanabe, K.; Tabuchi, S.; Watanabe, T.; Satoh, K. Nonenzymatic derived lipid peroxide, 8-iso-PGF2 alpha, participates in the pathogenesis of delayed cerebral vasospasm in a canine SAH model. *Neurol. Res.* **2002**, *24*, 301–306. [CrossRef] [PubMed]
134. Smeda, J.S.; Daneshtalab, N. The effects of poststroke captopril and losartan treatment on cerebral blood flow autoregulation in SHRsp with hemorrhagic stroke. *J. Cereb. Blood Flow Metab.* **2011**, *31*, 476–485. [CrossRef] [PubMed]
135. Tchekalarova, J.D.; Ivanova, N.M.; Pechlivanova, D.M.; Atanasovo, D.; Lazarov, N.; Kortenska, L.; Mitreva, R.; Lozanov, V.; Stoynev, A. Antiepileptogenic and neuroprotective effects of losartan in kainate model of temporal lobe epilepsy. *Pharmacol. Biochem. Behav.* **2014**, *127*, 27–36. [CrossRef] [PubMed]

136. Sun, H.; Wu, H.; Yu, X.; Zhang, G.; Zhang, R.; Zhan, S.; Wang, H.; Bu, N.; Ma, X.; Li, Y. Angiotensin II and its receptor in activated microglia enhanced neuronal loss and cognitive impairment following pilocarpine-induced status epilepticus. *Mol. Cell Neurosci.* **2015**, *65*, 58–67. [CrossRef]
137. Tchekalarova, J.D.; Ivanova, N.; Atanasova, D.; Pechlivanova, D.M.; Lazarov, N.; Kortenska, L.; Mitreva, R.; Lozanov, V.; Stoynev, A. Long-Term Treatment with Losartan Attenuates Seizure Activity and Neuronal Damage Without Affecting Behavioral Changes in a Model of Co-morbid Hypertension and Epilepsy. *Cell Mol. Neurobiol.* **2016**, *36*, 927–941. [CrossRef]
138. Nozaki, T.; Ura, H.; Takumi, I.; Kobayashi, S.; Maru, E.; Morita, A. The angiotensin II type I receptor antagonist losartan retards amygdala kindling-induced epileptogenesis. *Brain Res.* **2018**, *1694*, 121–128. [CrossRef]
139. Biancardi, V.C.; Stranahan, A.M.; Krause, E.G.; de Kloet, A.D.; Stern, J.E. Cross talk between AT1 receptors and Toll-like receptor 4 in microglia contributes to angiotensin II-derived ROS production in the hypothalamic paraventricular nucleus. *Am. J. Physiol. Heart Circ. Physiol.* **2016**, *310*, H404–H415. [CrossRef]
140. Maeso, R.; Rodrigo, E.; Munoz-Garcia, R.; Navarro-Cid, J.; Ruilope, L.M.; Lahera, V.; Cachofeiro, V. Losartan reduces constrictor responses to endothelin-1 and the thromboxane A2 analogue in aortic rings from spontaneously hypertensive rats: Role of nitric oxide. *J. Hypertens.* **1997**, *15*, 1677–1684. [CrossRef]
141. Guan, W.; Kozak, A.; El-Remessy, A.B.; Johnson, M.H.; Pillai, B.A.; Fagan, S.C. Acute treatment with candesartan reduces early injury after permanent middle cerebral artery occlusion. *Transl. Stroke Res.* **2011**, *2*, 179–185. [CrossRef] [PubMed]
142. Oku, N.; Kitagawa, K.; Imaizumi, M.; Takasawa, M.; Piao, R.; Kimura, Y.; Kajimoto, K.; Matsumoto, M.; Hori, M.; Hatazawa, J. Hemodynamic influences of losartan on the brain in hypertensive patients. *Hypertens. Res.* **2005**, *28*, 43–49. [CrossRef] [PubMed]
143. Habashi, J.P.; Judge, D.P.; Holm, T.M.; Cohn, R.D.; Loeys, B.L.; Cooper, T.K.; Myers, L.; Klein, E.C.; Liu, G.; Calvi, C. Losartan, an AT1 antagonist, prevents aortic aneurysm in a mouse model of Marfan syndrome. *Science* **2006**, *312*, 117–121. [CrossRef] [PubMed]
144. Povlsen, G.K.; Waldsee, R.; Ahnstedt, H.; Kristiansen, K.A.; Johansen, F.F.; Edvinsson, L. In vivo experimental stroke and in vitro organ culture induce similar changes in vasoconstrictor receptors and intracellular calcium handling in rat cerebral arteries. *Exp. Brain Res.* **2012**, *219*, 507–520. [CrossRef]
145. Vikman, P.; Beg, S.; Khurana, T.S.; Hansen-Schwartz, J.; Edvinsson, L. Gene expression and molecular changes in cerebral arteries following subarachnoid hemorrhage in the rat. *J. Neurosurg.* **2006**, *105*, 438–444. [CrossRef]
146. Dimitropoulou, C.; Chatterjee, A.; McCloud, L.; Yetik-Anacak, G.; Catravas, J.D. Angiotensin, bradykinin and the endothelium. In *Handbook of Experimental Pharmacology*; Springer: New York, NY, USA, 2006; Volume 176, pp. 255–294.
147. Tirapelli, C.R.; Bonaventura, D.; Tirapelli, L.F.; de Oliveira, A.M. Mechanisms underlying the vascular actions of endothelin 1, angiotensin II and bradykinin in the rat carotid. *Pharmacology* **2009**, *84*, 111–126. [CrossRef]
148. Mehta, P.K.; Griendling, K.K. Angiotensin II cell signaling: Physiological and pathological effects in the cardiovascular system. *Am. J. Physiol. Cell Physiol.* **2007**, *292*, C82–C97. [CrossRef]
149. Arai, H.; Hori, S.; Aramori, I.; Ohkubo, H.; Nakanishi, S. Cloning and expression of a cDNA encoding an endothelin receptor. *Nature* **1990**, *348*, 730–732. [CrossRef]
150. Toda, N.; Miyazaki, M. Angiotensin-induced relaxation in isolated dog renal and cerebral arteries. *Am. J. Physiol.* **1981**, *240*, H247–H254. [CrossRef]
151. Tsutsumi, Y.; Matsubara, H.; Masaki, H.; Kurihara, H.; Murasawa, S.; Takai, S.; Miyazaki, M.; Nozawa, Y.; Ozono, R.; Nakagawa, K.; et al. Angiotensin II type 2 receptor overexpression activates the vascular kinin system and causes vasodilation. *J. Clin. Investig.* **1999**, *104*, 925–935. [CrossRef]
152. Abassi, Z.A.; Klein, H.; Golomb, E.; Keiser, H.R. Regulation of the urinary excretion of endothelin in the rat. *Am. J. Hypertens.* **1993**, *6*, 453–457. [CrossRef] [PubMed]
153. Brunner, F.; Kukovetz, W.R. Postischemic antiarrhythmic effects of angiotensin-converting enzyme inhibitors. Role of suppression of endogenous endothelin secretion. *Circulation* **1996**, *94*, 1752–1761. [CrossRef] [PubMed]
154. Chua, B.H.; Chua, C.C.; Diglio, C.A.; Siu, B.B. Regulation of endothelin-1 mRNA by angiotensin II in rat heart endothelial cells. *Biochim. Biophys. Acta* **1993**, *1178*, 201–206. [CrossRef]

155. Dohi, Y.; Hahn, A.W.; Boulanger, C.M.; Buhler, F.R.; Luscher, T.F. Endothelin stimulated by angiotensin II augments contractility of spontaneously hypertensive rat resistance arteries. *Hypertension* **1992**, *19*, 131–137. [CrossRef]
156. Kohno, M.; Horio, T.; Ikeda, M.; Yokokawa, K.; Fukui, T.; Yasunari, K.; Kurihara, N.; Takeda, T. Angiotensin II stimulates endothelin-1 secretion in cultured rat mesangial cells. *Kidney Int.* **1992**, *42*, 860–866. [CrossRef]
157. Saavedra, J.M.; Benicky, J.; Zhou, J. Mechanisms of the Anti-Ischemic Effect of Angiotensin II AT(1) Receptor Antagonists in the Brain. *Cell Mol. Neurobiol.* **2006**, *26*, 1099–1111. [CrossRef]

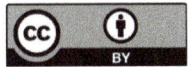 © 2020 by the authors. Licensee MDPI, Basel, Switzerland. This article is an open access article distributed under the terms and conditions of the Creative Commons Attribution (CC BY) license (http://creativecommons.org/licenses/by/4.0/).

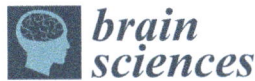 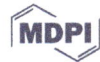

Review

Preclinical Intracranial Aneurysm Models: A Systematic Review

Fabio Strange [1,2,*], Basil E Grüter [1,2], Javier Fandino [1,2] and Serge Marbacher [1,2]

1   Department of Neurosurgery, 5001 Kantonsspital Aarau, Switzerland; basil.grueter@ksa.ch (B.E.G.); javier.fandino@ksa.ch (J.F.); serge.marbacher@ksa.ch (S.M.)
2   Cerebrovascular Research Group, Department for BioMedical Research, University of Bern, 3008 Bern, Switzerland
*   Correspondence: fabio.strange@ksa.ch

Received: 31 January 2020; Accepted: 23 February 2020; Published: 27 February 2020

Abstract: Intracranial aneurysms (IA) are characterized by weakened cerebral vessel walls that may lead to rupture and subarachnoid hemorrhage. The mechanisms behind their formation and progression are yet unclear and warrant preclinical studies. This systematic review aims to provide a comprehensive, systematic overview of available animal models for the study of IA pathobiology. We conducted a systematic literature search using the PubMed database to identify preclinical studies employing IA animal models. Suitable articles were selected based on predefined eligibility criteria following the Preferred Reporting Items for Systematic Reviews and Meta-Analyses (PRISMA) guidelines. Included studies were reviewed and categorized according to the experimental animal and aneurysm model. Of 4266 returned results, 3930 articles were excluded based on the title and/or abstract and further articles after screening the full text, leaving 123 studies for detailed analysis. A total of 20 different models were found in rats (nine), mice (five), rabbits (four), and dogs (two). Rat models constituted the most frequently employed intracranial experimental aneurysm model (79 studies), followed by mice (31 studies), rabbits (12 studies), and two studies in dogs. The most common techniques to induce cerebral aneurysms were surgical ligation of the common carotid artery with subsequent induction of hypertension by ligation of the renal arteries, followed by elastase-induced creation of IAs in combination with corticosterone- or angiotensin-induced hypertension. This review provides a comprehensive summary of the multitude of available IA models to study various aspects of aneurysm formation, growth, and rupture. It will serve as a useful reference for researchers by facilitating the selection of the most appropriate model and technique to answer their scientific question.

Keywords: animal model; aneurysm; cerebral aneurysm; intracranial aneurysm

1. Introduction

Intracranial aneurysm (IA) refers to an outward bulging of the arterial wall and is a serious cerebrovascular disease with a high morbidity and mortality [1]. It is characterized by a chronic inflammation and weakening of the arterial walls [2]. The prognosis of IA is poor, due to a rupture of the lesions and the ensuing subarachnoid hemorrhage that is responsible for the high number of IA-induced fatalities. Even though the prevalence of IA is high (2–8% [3]), there is currently no proven therapy that achieves stabilization and prevention of rupture. Most IA patients are treated conservatively, and only those with a presumably high risk of IA rupture (depending on the IA size, smoking status and location [4]) undergo occlusion [5]. The successful development and implementation of therapeutic strategies to avoid IA formation, and particularly subarachnoid hemorrhage, is hence of clinical importance. A prerequisite for any effective therapy is a better understanding of IA pathobiology. Moreover, both the efficacy and potential side effects of a novel drug need to be carefully assessed before it may be administered to IA patients, requiring a thorough preclinical investigation that precedes the translation in the clinical practice. Since the natural formation of IA is rare in animals, techniques to artificially induce IA in experimental animals have been developed. Researchers interested in the study of IA pathobiology are now facing a broad variety of animal models to choose from [6]. These involve models in different species and numerous variations of the originally developed methods, which differ in their comparability to human IAs, the complexity of the methodology, and the questions that can be answered. Furthermore, the technique to induce hypertension constitutes a common variation of the initial, well-established models. The large volume of available models may complicate the selection of the appropriate model for the respective research question. We therefore set out to compile systematic literature review on available IA animal models as a comprehensive reference for researchers planning to employ such a model in their investigations. We discuss advantages and disadvantages of each model and address considerations regarding the species and method of choice.

2. Materials and Methods

A systematic literature search in the Medline/PubMed database was conducted to identify preclinical studies using IA animal models. The search was performed on November 31, 2017 with the keywords "mice", "rat", "rabbit", "dog", and "swine" in combination with "aneurysm" using the Boolean operator [AND]. Studies on primates were excluded due to their limited ethical justifiability. The search was restricted to "animals". Two investigators (SM and FS) independently screened titles and abstracts and selected suitable studies based on predefined eligibility criteria following the Preferred Reporting Items for Systematic Reviews and Meta-Analyses (PRISMA) [7]. The final articles to be included were selected based on the full text of eligible studies. Discrepancies in the study selection were discussed with all authors and a consensus was reached. Included studies were reviewed and categorized according to the experimental animal used and the aneurysm model employed.

The eligibility criteria were as follows: (1) in vivo IA model in the experimental species rat, mouse, rabbit, dog, and swine; (2) English language; (3) original research article (reviews, letters, and editorials were excluded).

The following data were extracted from eligible full text articles: (1) authors and year of publication; (2) study question and main conclusion; (3) animal species; (4) method to create IA; (5) IA location; and (6) time until sacrifice/study duration.

The same method to generate IA in different species was considered a separate model. Modifications of an existing model such as extension of the technique itself or of significant accessory techniques (e.g., induction of hypertension by renal artery (RA) ligation) were also categorized as individual models.

3. Results

The literature searches initially returned 4264 articles, of which 3930 were excluded after title and/or abstract screening because they did not meet the eligibility criteria. A further 211 articles were excluded after screening the full text due to one or more of the following reasons: duplicate article, article was withdrawn, the type of article differed from an original research study such as a review, letter or comment, or the article was written in a language other than English. This strategy left 123 studies for a detailed analysis (Figure 1).

A total of 20 different models were identified based on the technique to create IA (common carotid artery (CCA) ligation (unilateral or bilateral), (renal artery [RA] ligation [unilateral or bilateral], elastase injection [with or without CCA ligation] and experimental species [rat, mouse, rabbit, dog])) (Table 1). Only those modifications that affected the ligation surgery (i.e., RA ligation or not) were considered as separate models. Smaller variations to the induction of hypertension (i.e., different NaCl concentrations, β-aminopropionitrile monofumarate (BAPN) or estrogen depletion) were not considered as novel models. Of the identified distinct models, 9 different models were used in rats, 5 in mice, 4 in rabbits, and 2 in dogs (see Table 1 for detailed listing of studies according to the IA model).

The identified IA animal models were assigned to one of the following main categories: (1) CCA ligation with concomitant RA ligation, (2) CCA ligation only, (3) elastase injection, (4) elastase injection and CCA ligation, or (5) another model.

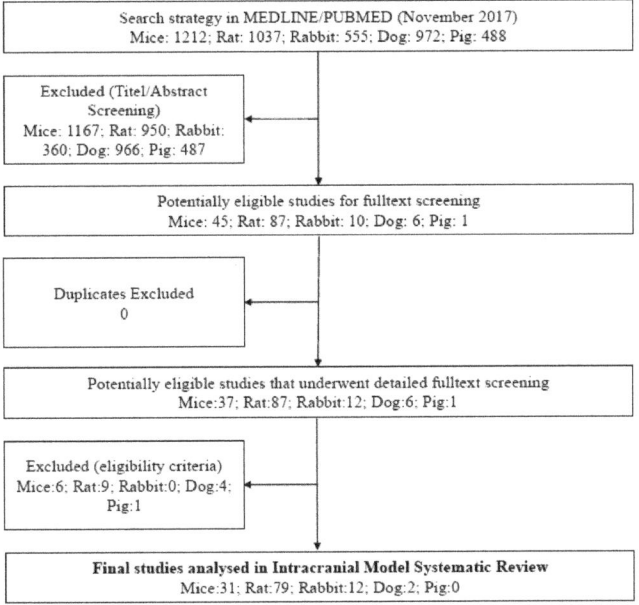

Figure 1. Preferred Reporting Items for Systematic Reviews and Meta-Analyses (PRISMA) flow chart for study selection.

Table 1. Overview of included studies. The most commonly used model in rats was common carotid artery (CCA) ligation and renal artery (RA) ligation, in mice elastase injection, and in rabbits CCA ligation.

Category	Subcategory	References
CCA ligation	Unilateral CCA ligation	Rat: Alvarez et al. 1986 [8], Cai et al. 2012 [9], Coutard et al. 2000 [10], Hahimoto et al. 1978 [11], 1979a [12], 1979b [13], 1980 [14], Ishibashi et al. 2012 [15], Kaufmann et al. 2006 [16], Matsushita et al. 2012 [17], Suzuki et al. 1980 [18], Roda et al. 1988 [19], Xu et al. 2011a [20], 2011b [21].
		Mouse: Abruzzo et al. 2007 [22]
		Rabbit: Dai et al. 2013 [23], Gao et al. 2008 [24]
	Bilateral CCA ligation	Rat: Tutino et al. 2016 [25]
		Rabbit: Dolan et al. 2013 [26], Kolega et al. 2011 [27], Li et al. 2014 [28], Liaw et al. 2014 [29], Mandelbaum et al. 2013 [30], Metaxa et al. 2010 [31], Tutino et al. 2014 [32], 2015 [33]
CCA ligation and RA ligation	Unilateral RA ligation	Rat: Aoki 2007 [34], 2014 [35], Coutard et al. 1997 [36], Fukuda et al. 2014 [37], Ikedo et al. 2017 [38], Miyata et al. 2017 [39], Yamamoto et al. 2017 [40]
		Mouse: Aoki et al. 2007 [34], 2017, Moriwaki et al. 2006 [41]
		Rabbit: Gao et al. 2008 [24]
	Bilateral RA ligation	Rat: Alvarez and Roda 1986 [8], Aoki et al. 2007a [42], 2007b [43], 2008a [44], 2008b [45], 2008c [46], 2008d [47], 2009 [48], 2010a [49], 2010b [50], 2011 [51], 2012 [52], 2017a [53], 2017b [54], Eldawoody et al. 2009 [55], Futami et al. 1995a [56], 1995b [57], 1998 [58], Guo et al. 2016 [59], Hazama et al. 1986 [60], Ishibashi et al. 2010 [61], Jamous et al. 2005a [62], 2005b [63], 2005c [64], 2007 [65], Kang et al. 1990 [66], Kim et al. 1988 [67], Kimura et al. 2010 [69], Kojima et al. 1986 [70], Kondo et al. 1997 [71], 1998 [72], Korai et al. 2016 [73], Li et al. 2014 [74], 2015 [75], Maekawa et al. 2017 [76], Miyamoto et al. 2017 [77], Nagata et al. 1979 [78], 1980 [79], 1981 [80], Nakatani et al. 1993 [81], Sadamasa et al. 2007 [82], 2008 [83], Tada et al. 2010 [84], 2011 [85], Tamura et al. 2009 [86], Yagi et al. 2010 [87], Yamazoe et al. 1990 [88], Yokoi et al. 2014 [89], Wu et al. 2016 [90], Zhou et al. 1985 [91]
		Mouse: Sadamasa et al. 2003 [92]
		Rat: Zhao et al. 2015 [93]
	Elastase injection	Mouse: Chalouhi et al. 2016 [94], Chu et al. 2015 [95], Hasan et al. 2015 [96], Kanematsu et al. 2011 [97], Kuwabara et al. 2017 [98], Labeyrie et al. 2017 [99], Lee et al. 2016 [100], Liu et al. 2016 [101], 2017 [102], Makino et al. 2012 [103], 2015 [104], Nuki et al. 2009 [105], Pena Silva et al. 2014 [106], 2015 [107], Shimada et al. 2015a [108], 2015b [109], Tada et al. 2014a [110], 2014b [111], 2014c [112], Wada et al. 2014 [113], Zhang et al. 2015 [114]
		Rabbit: Dai et al. 2010 [115], Yasuda et al. 2005 [116]
	Elastase injection and CCA ligation	Mouse: Hoh et al. 2014 [117], Hosaka et al. 2014 [118], 2017 [119], Nowicki et al. 2017 [120]
Other	Deoxycorticosterone/hypertension	Lee et al. 1978 [121] (rat)
	Eplerenone	Tada et al. 2009 [122] (rat)
	Copper deficiency	Jung et al. 2016 [123] (rat)
	CaCl2	Bo et al. 2017 [124] (rat)
	Coating of internal carotid artery	Ebina et al. 1984 [125] (dog)
	Venous pouch or venous patch	Nishikawa et al. 1977 [126] (dog)

The most common technique to induce cerebral aneurysms was surgical ligation of the CCA and/or the RA with concomitant induction of hypertension (64 studies), followed by CCA ligation without RA manipulation (24 studies) and elastase-induced creation of IAs in combination with corticosterone- or angiotensin II-induced hypertension (24 studies, see Table 2 for an overview of IA model by experimental animal). Thirteen studies employed alternative methods to create IA. Of the models using CCA ligation, unilateral ligation of the left CCA was performed in most models, but ligation of the right CCA or bilateral ligation was also common. CCA ligation was most common in rats and rabbits, whereas the elastase method was used in most mouse models. The category "other models" included IA creation by deoxycorticosterone administration [121], eplerenone administration [122], induction of copper deficiency [123], CaCl$_2$ treatment [124], coating of the internal carotid artery [125], with one study for each of these models.

Table 2. Number of aneurysm type per species in the included studies. The vast majority (76%) of studies in rats used a combined CCA ligation and RA ligation model, whereas most mouse studies (68%) used an Elastase only model. CCA = common carotid artery; RA = renal artery.

Species	Total No. of Studies Analyzed	CCA Ligation and RA Ligation	CCA Ligation Only	Elastase Only	Elastase and CCA Ligation	Other
Mice	31	4	1	21	4	-
Rats	79	60	13	1	-	5
Rabbits	21	-	10	1	1	-
Dogs	2	-	-	-	-	2
Overall	133	64	24	22	5	6

Most of the assessed studies used rats for their animal model (79 studies), followed by mice (31 studies), and rabbits (12 studies). Only two studies were performed in dogs. Almost half of the mouse models were employed in transgenic animals [22,41,43,53,92,95,96,99,102,105,106,109,112,114,127].

The most frequent variation of the original models was modification of the technique to induce hypertension rather than of the IA creation technique itself. Hypertension was typically achieved by using one or a combination of RA ligation, high salt diet, or deoxycorticosterone administration (Table 3). A further variation of the original CCA model was omission of BAPN administration to inhibit cross-linking of collagen and elastin, which was contraindicated depending on certain research questions [56].

Table 3. Mean time of aneurysm formation in months (range).

Species	CCA Ligation and RA Ligation	CCA Ligation Only	Elastase Only	Elastase and CCA Ligation	Other
Mice (31)	3,4 (0,5–5)	13 (0)	0,53 (0,17–1)	0,43 (0,1–0,75)	-
Rats (79)	2,28 (0,17–12)	2,49 (0,25–12)	1,25 (0)	-	1,83 (1–2,5)
Rabbits (12)	3,0	2,59 (0,17–6)	1,5 (1–2)	-	-
Dogs (2)	-	-	-	-	0,68 (0,35–1)
Overall	2,38 (0,17–12)	2,53 (0,17–13)	0,65 (0,17–2)	0,43 (0,1–0,75)	1,37 (0,35–2,5)

The study duration before sacrifice and assessment of the animal varied between a few weeks [38,105] and a year [16,71], but typically lasted 1 to 3 months.

4. Discussion

By conducting a comprehensive systematic review of the literature, we achieved categorization of the IA animal models available to date and developed an overview that should facilitate the choice of the experimental animal and most appropriate technique for researchers interested in IA pathobiology. Surgical ligation of the CCA and elastase-induced weakening of the arterial vessel wall was identified as the predominant techniques to create IA in experimental animals. A brief discussion of the advantages and disadvantages of each of these categories follows.

General Considerations

Ethics: Animal ethics regulations have become increasingly strict in recent years in terms of the species of animal and required numbers to be used in experimental studies. Studies on animals that raise particular ethical concerns, such as those conducted in dogs, primates and swine, are likely to face more obstacles throughout the animal ethics approval process, which may delay the conduction of the study or entirely prevent its completion. Small animals that are more commonly used in research such as rats and mice appear often more feasible than those in large animals, yet the study needs to be carefully designed to ensure statistically feasible justification of the required animal numbers, particularly in cases where it is unknown if and for how long the animals will survive the experiment, as is the case for all intracranial animal models.

Costs: Similar to the ethical concerns, the maintenance and housing of large animals can infer tremendous costs on the researcher. In addition, the potential costs need to consider the duration of the experiments, as some of the aneurysm models last for more than three months, during which time the animals need to be housed and likely monitored daily, which results in additional costs for animal care personnel and veterinarians.

Reliability: Most intracranial aneurysm models are conducted in rats by unilateral CCA ligation and concomitant RA ligation (Table 2). This can be attributed to the reliability of such a model in producing aneurysms in the majority of experimental animals in a comparatively very short period of time of less than three months (Table 3). These models are so reliable because they are based on a long history of refinement and modifications, Table S1 tweaking the technique to a point where aneurysm development is guaranteed. An even faster generation of aneurysms is observed in the elastase model in mice, yet it appears that this model does not work well in rats, therefore one needs to balance the time of formation with the most suitable species for the experiment. The best model clearly depends on the research question to be answered. If aneurysm growth is the main factor to be investigated, surgical ligation models are to be favored over others, as the procedure allows for variation in the size of the aneurysm and may generate very large aneurysms in the animals. In turn, if aneurysm rupture is the center of the investigation, the surgical model needs to be combined with a treatment to induce hypertension such as administering NaCl in the drinking water or implanting a salt pellet with dosed release. Alternatively, the elastase model is frequently used in mechanistic and pharmacological aneurysm rupture studies as it generates ruptures through subarachnoid hemorrhages within a relatively short period of time (one month).

Ligation of the CCA, with or without concomitant RA ligation: This original model first described in the 1970s by Hashimoto et al. [11] and Nagata et al. [78] involves unilateral ligation of the CCA, for which most frequently the left CCA is manipulated. The ligation is accompanied by additional induction of hypertension using either ligation of one or both RAs, feeding of a high salt diet, administration of deoxycorticosterone, or a combination of these parameters (Table 4). In order to increase the animal's susceptibility to IA formation and shortening of the IA induction time, CCA ligation may be combined with administration of β-aminopropionitrile, a lathyrogen that inhibits the cross-linking of collagen and elastin, or with estrogen depletion achieved by oophorectomy to compromise endothelial cell function and NO (nitrogen oxide) release. Most rat models employ unilateral CCA ligation combined with bilateral RA ligation and a high salt diet, while in rabbits, both CCAs are often ligated without any further means of inducing hypertension. In mice, unilateral CCA ligation was complemented by contralateral ligation of one RA.

Table 4. Variations to established IA models pertaining to the technique to induce hypertension and weaken vessel walls.

Technique	Purpose	Number of Studies	Number of Species
RA ligation, unilateral	Hypertension	12	3
RA ligation, bilateral	Hypertension	52	2
High NaCl diet (1% or 8%)	Hypertension	68	3
Deoxycorticosterone administration	Hypertension	15	3
Angiotensin II	Hypertension	13	1
β-aminopropionitrile administration (0.12%)	Weakening of vessel walls	36	2
Estrogen depletion/oophorectomy	Weakening of vessel walls	12	3

Note: several methods may have been used concomitantly in the same animal or study. High NaCl diet followed by bilateral RA ligation were the most commonly used techniques. RA = renal artery; NaCl = sodium chloride.

The major advantage of this model is that is has been well established and refined for decades and has been shown to reliably induce IA in rats, mice and rabbits. It has been employed to answer a broad variety of research questions, ranging from the contribution of isolated factors to aneurysm formation to the success of therapeutic agents in the prevention and treatment of IAs.

Elastase treatment: As an alternative to the classical vessel ligation model, several more recent studies employ the injection of elastase into the cerebrospinal fluid or a common artery to disrupt the elastic lamina and thereby weaken the vessel walls. Concomitant induction of hypertension is achieved by continuous administration of angiotensin II with the aid of an implanted osmotic mini-pump, or by a combined administration of a high salt diet and deoxycorticosterone. This model is employed in mice and rabbits but rarely in rats. It accomplishes creation of large aneurysms within a relatively short study period. In a few models, both the injection of elastase and artery ligation were performed.

Elastase treatment and ligation of the CCA: IA generation by elastase injection may be supported by concomitant ligation of the CCA. We identified only four studies that employed this model, and mice were the only experimental animal used. Hence, this model has apparently not been tested in other experimental animals. Of note, this model involved the shortest study period, with IA creation achieved several days following the induction and a mean generation time of less than half a month (Figure 2, Table 3).

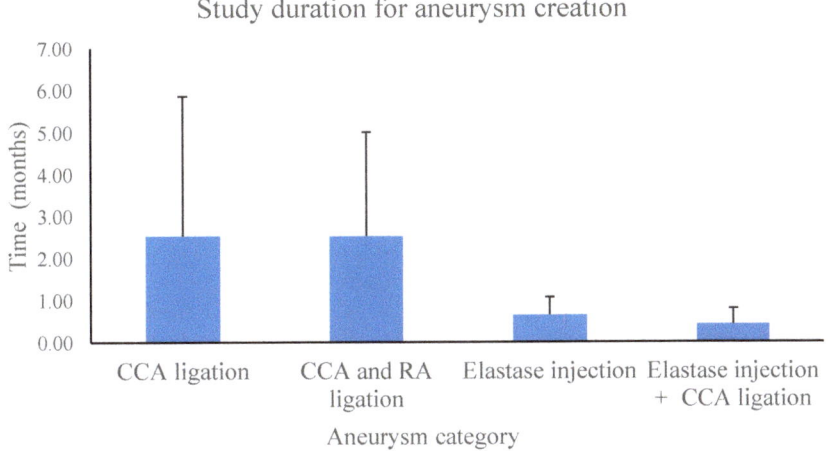

Figure 2. Meta-analysis of all intracranial aneurysm models to determine the shortest required study period for intracranial aneurysm (IA) generation. Common carotid artery (CA) ligation alone or in combination with renal artery (RA) ligation typically involved a period of several months, while intracranial aneurysms could be created by elastase injection with or without common carotid artery ligation in one month or less. Bars indicate mean + SD.

Once the type of IA model has been identified, the choice of experimental animal species must be considered, considering that the situation in the animal should be comparable to human IA pathophysiology. Most IA models are performed in small animals such as rats and mice. A limitation of all models is that IA do not easily develop spontaneously in animals and hence always constitute an artificially induced entity.

Certain models apparently work better in one species than the other [25]. The total study duration needs to be estimated; e.g., how long does it take to induce an aneurysm in an animal, and is this duration feasible for the study setting? We performed a meta-analysis of all selected studies with regards to the time it took to develop IAs following the induction (Figure 2, Table 3). Elastase injection alone (0.65 ± 0.43 months), or in combination with CCA ligation (0.43 ± 0.38 months), required a shorter time for IA generation than CCA alone (2.53 ± 3.33 months) or in combination with RA ligation (2.38 ± 2.48 months; Figure 2). The shortest study period was observed in a mouse model with elastase injection (0.1 month), while a model with CCA ligation in mice (13 months) took the longest (Table 3).

In addition, the number of animals that can be used is determined by the breeding time, housing space and animal care cost, and is to be carefully considered to obtain an animal number that can reach statistical significance (Collaborative Approach to Meta-Analysis and Review of Animal Data from Experimental Studies/CAMARADES [128]). Furthermore, different strains of the same species may differ in their susceptibility to IA formation [36]. Practical aspects also play a role in the species choice, such as the space that is required for the surgery (e.g., can it be done in a designated laboratory space or is an operating theater required) and the level of difficulty of the surgery itself (e.g., is an anesthesiologist required, how technically challenging is the surgery). The estimation of whether the respective research question can be appropriately answered with the experimental animal species is of utmost importance. For example, if the contribution of an isolated factor is to be investigated, a strain with a genetic knockdown of the gene of choice may be useful, which then renders a genetic mouse model the most suitable choice. Animal ethics need to be considered as well, as canine studies are not only expensive but also ethically challenging. Concerns over the ethical treatment of animals led to the development of the "3R principle" that aims to replace, reduce, or refine experiments using experimental animals; owing to this principle, primates are rarely used these days as research models. For this reason, we did not extend the scope of the present review to this species as they are only employed in exceptional cases. Advantages and disadvantages of each model are discussed as follows.

Rats: The major advantage of using rats as an experimental model is the availability of a well-established model that works well and has been described in detail with slight variations for decades. CCA ligation in combination with RA ligation appears to be the gold standard for IA creation, and the investigator can make a well informed choice of the experimental specifications due to the plethora of available literature. Furthermore, rats are commonly used experimental animals, are easily available, instill only moderate costs for housing and feed, and breed fast, making it possible to conduct studies with many animals to reach statistical significance. Moreover, anesthetic techniques are well established in this species and can be easily maintained in a typical research laboratory without the need for a designated operating theater or a veterinary anesthesiologist. The surgery is manageable (not as small as in the mouse but still comparable to humans) and may be relatively easily learned by a new scientist entering the field. The disadvantage of using rats is that the elastase model apparently does not work as well in rats as in mice, and neither does bilateral CCA ligation should it be required. In addition, although genetic knockout models in rats are available, they generate considerably higher costs compared to such models in mice.

Mice: Mice share the same practical advantages as rats, in that their housing and feed is comparatively cheap, they breed fast, and are well maintained during surgery on basic anesthetic techniques. The major advantage of using mice as an experimental model is the possibility to investigate an isolated factor that may contribute to IA formation or protect from it in transgenic animals, be it knockout mouse models or animals overexpressing certain genes. Particularly, the elastase model is well established in mice, and the CCA ligation model has also been successfully employed in this species. A disadvantage of using mice may be the somewhat delicate surgery on very small vessels, which could require some practice to achieve an optimum outcome.

Rabbits: Bilateral CCA ligation is particularly well established in rabbits and appears to work better in this species than in rats. None of the studies included in this review employed RA ligation in rabbits, and only one study described the elastase model. In terms of practicability, rabbits incur a somewhat larger cost for housing than rats and mice as they require more space. It may also not be possible to conduct surgery on these animals in any regular laboratory space, but rather an operating theater might be required.

Dogs: We identified only two studies using distinct IA models in dogs as experimental animals, both of which were dated (1977 and 1984). It has to be noted that angiography is an investigative technique available for dogs that does not require sacrifice of the animal. Nevertheless, it appears that both the much more extensive cost in combination with ethical considerations does not render this species a model that can be routinely employed. The same holds true for swine and primates as experimental animals to create IAs. Few studies exist that use large species to produce IAs. The few published studies are considered historical series rather than models that are still in use today. Considering ethical concerns, it is unlikely that these species/models will gain importance in the future.

5. Conclusions

We provide a categorization of available IA animal models and thereby present a tool to guide researchers entering the field of aneurysm pathobiology. The best choice of a specific IA model strongly depends on the individual research question and numerous other factors such as the primary endpoint, available resources (e.g., expenses for animal housing and breeding, space for surgical procedures, need for veterinary anesthesiologist), and time frame for IA initiation, growth, and rupture (weeks to months).

Supplementary Materials: The following are available online at http://www.mdpi.com/2076-3425/10/3/134/s1, Table S1: Incidence of Aneurysm development.

Author Contributions: F.S. and S.M.: design of the systematic review, collection and analysis of data, drafting the manuscript; F.S., S.M., B.E.G. and J.F.: critical revision of the first draft; all of the authors: critical revision of the final manuscript. All authors have read and agreed to the published version of the manuscript.

Funding: This study was supported by a research grant from the Kantonsspital Aarau, Aarau, Switzerland (FR 1400.000.054).

Conflicts of Interest: The authors declare no conflict of interest.

References

1. Etminan, N.; Rinkel, G.J. Unruptured intracranial aneurysms: Development, rupture and preventive management. *Nat. Rev. Neurol.* **2016**, *12*, 699–713. [CrossRef] [PubMed]
2. Fukuda, M.; Aoki, T. Molecular basis for intracranial aneurysm formation. *Acta Neurochir. Suppl.* **2015**, *120*, 13–15. [CrossRef] [PubMed]
3. Vlak, M.H.; Algra, A.; Brandenburg, R.; Rinkel, G.J. Prevalence of unruptured intracranial aneurysms, with emphasis on sex, age, comorbidity, country, and time period: A systematic review and meta-analysis. *Lancet Neurol.* **2011**, *10*, 626–636. [CrossRef]
4. Brinjikji, W.; Pereira, V.M.; Khumtong, R.; Kostensky, A.; Tymianski, M.; Krings, T.; Radovanovich, I. PHASES and ELAPSS scores are associated with aneurysm growth: A study of 431 unruptured intracranial aneurysms. *World Neurosurg.* **2018**, *114*, e425–e432. [CrossRef] [PubMed]
5. Diaz, O.; Rangel-Castilla, L. Endovascular treatment of intracranial aneurysms. *Handb. Clin. Neurol.* **2016**, *136*, 1303–1309. [CrossRef]
6. Bouzeghrane, F.; Naggara, O.; Kallmes, D.F.; Berenstein, A.; Raymond, J.; International Consortium of Neuro Endovascular Centres. In vivo experimental intracranial aneurysm models: A systematic review. *AJNR Am. J. Neuroradiol.* **2010**, *31*, 418–423. [CrossRef]

7. Moher, D.; Liberati, A.; Tetzlaff, J.; Altman, D.G.; Group, P. Preferred reporting items for systematic reviews and meta-analyses: The PRISMA statement. *Int. J. Surg.* **2010**, *8*, 336–341. [CrossRef]
8. Alvarez, F.; Roda, J.M. Experimental model for induction of cerebral aneurysms in rats. *J. Neurosurg.* **1986**, *65*, 398–400. [CrossRef]
9. Cai, J.; He, C.; Yuan, F.; Chen, L.; Ling, F. A novel haemodynamic cerebral aneurysm model of rats with normal blood pressure. *J. Clin. Neurosci.* **2012**, *19*, 135–138. [CrossRef]
10. Coutard, M.; Huang, W.; Osborne-Pellegrin, M. Heritability of intracerebral hemorrhagic lesions and cerebral aneurysms in the rat. *Stroke* **2000**, *31*, 2678–2684. [CrossRef]
11. Hashimoto, N.; Handa, H.; Hazama, F. Experimentally induced cerebral aneurysms in rats. *Surg. Neurol.* **1978**, *10*, 3–8. [PubMed]
12. Hashimoto, N.; Handa, H.; Hazama, F. Experimentally induced cerebral aneurysms in rats: Part II. *Surg. Neurol.* **1979**, *11*, 243–246. [PubMed]
13. Hashimoto, N.; Handa, H.; Hazama, F. Experimentally induced cerebral aneurysms in rats: Part III. Pathology. *Surg. Neurol.* **1979**, *11*, 299–304. [PubMed]
14. Hashimoto, N.; Handa, H.; Nagata, I.; Hazama, F. Experimentally induced cerebral aneurysms in rats: Part V. Relation of hemodynamics in the circle of Willis to formation of aneurysms. *Surg. Neurol.* **1980**, *13*, 41–45.
15. Ishibashi, R.; Aoki, T.; Nishimura, M.; Miyamoto, S. Imidapril inhibits cerebral aneurysm formation in an angiotensin-converting enzyme-independent and matrix metalloproteinase-9-dependent manner. *Neurosurgery* **2012**, *70*, 722–730. [CrossRef]
16. Kaufmann, T.J.; Marx, W.F.; Kallmes, D.F. A failure of matrix metalloproteinase inhibition in the prevention of rat intracranial aneurysm formation. *Neuroradiology* **2006**, *48*, 190–195. [CrossRef]
17. Matsushita, N.; Kitazato, K.T.; Tada, Y.; Sumiyoshi, M.; Shimada, K.; Yagi, K.; Kanematsu, Y.; Satomi, J.; Nagahiro, S. Increase in body Na+/water ratio is associated with cerebral aneurysm formation in oophorectomized rats. *Hypertension* **2012**, *60*, 1309–1315. [CrossRef]
18. Suzuki, S.; Robertson, J.T.; White, R.P.; Stadlan, E.M.; Popoff, N. Experimental intracranial aneurysms in rats. A gross and microscopic study. *J. Neurosurg.* **1980**, *52*, 494–500. [CrossRef]
19. Roda, J.M.; Alvarez, F.; Garcia-Villalon, A.L.; Ruiz, M.R.; Gutierrez, M.; Garcia Blazquez, M. An increment in unilateral carotid blood flow produces cerebral aneurysms in rats. *Acta Neurochir. Suppl. (Wien)* **1988**, *43*, 189–192.
20. Xu, Y.; Tian, Y.; Wei, H.J.; Chen, J.; Dong, J.F.; Zacharek, A.; Zhang, J.N. Erythropoietin increases circulating endothelial progenitor cells and reduces the formation and progression of cerebral aneurysm in rats. *Neuroscience* **2011**, *181*, 292–299. [CrossRef]
21. Xu, Y.; Tian, Y.; Wei, H.J.; Dong, J.F.; Zhang, J.N. Methionine diet-induced hyperhomocysteinemia accelerates cerebral aneurysm formation in rats. *Neurosci. Lett.* **2011**, *494*, 139–144. [CrossRef] [PubMed]
22. Abruzzo, T.; Kendler, A.; Apkarian, R.; Workman, M.; Khoury, J.C.; Cloft, H.J. Cerebral aneurysm formation in nitric oxide synthase-3 knockout mice. *Curr. Neurovasc. Res.* **2007**, *4*, 161–169. [CrossRef] [PubMed]
23. Dai, D.; Ding, Y.H.; Kadirvel, R.; Rad, A.E.; Lewis, D.A.; Kallmes, D.F. Lack of aneurysm formation after carotid artery ligation in rabbits: A polymer MICROFIL(R) study. *Neuroradiology* **2013**, *55*, 65–70. [CrossRef] [PubMed]
24. Gao, L.; Hoi, Y.; Swartz, D.D.; Kolega, J.; Siddiqui, A.; Meng, H. Nascent aneurysm formation at the basilar terminus induced by hemodynamics. *Stroke* **2008**, *39*, 2085–2090. [CrossRef]
25. Tutino, V.M.; Liaw, N.; Spernyak, J.A.; Ionita, C.N.; Siddiqui, A.H.; Kolega, J.; Meng, H. Assessment of vascular geometry for bilateral carotid artery ligation to induce early basilar terminus aneurysmal remodeling in rats. *Curr. Neurovasc. Res.* **2016**, *13*, 82–92. [CrossRef] [PubMed]
26. Dolan, J.M.; Meng, H.; Sim, F.J.; Kolega, J. Differential gene expression by endothelial cells under positive and negative streamwise gradients of high wall shear stress. *Am. J. Physiol. Cell Physiol.* **2013**, *305*, C854–C866. [CrossRef]
27. Kolega, J.; Gao, L.; Mandelbaum, M.; Mocco, J.; Siddiqui, A.H.; Natarajan, S.K.; Meng, H. Cellular and molecular responses of the basilar terminus to hemodynamics during intracranial aneurysm initiation in a rabbit model. *J. Vasc. Res.* **2011**, *48*, 429–442. [CrossRef]
28. Li, M.H.; Li, P.G.; Huang, Q.L.; Ling, J. Endothelial injury preceding intracranial aneurysm formation in rabbits. *West Indian Med. J.* **2014**, *63*, 167–171. [CrossRef]

29. Liaw, N.; Fox, J.M.; Siddiqui, A.H.; Meng, H.; Kolega, J. Endothelial nitric oxide synthase and superoxide mediate hemodynamic initiation of intracranial aneurysms. *PLoS ONE* **2014**, *9*, e101721. [CrossRef]
30. Mandelbaum, M.; Kolega, J.; Dolan, J.M.; Siddiqui, A.H.; Meng, H. A critical role for proinflammatory behavior of smooth muscle cells in hemodynamic initiation of intracranial aneurysm. *PLoS ONE* **2013**, *8*, e74357. [CrossRef]
31. Metaxa, E.; Tremmel, M.; Natarajan, S.K.; Xiang, J.; Paluch, R.A.; Mandelbaum, M.; Siddiqui, A.H.; Kolega, J.; Mocco, J.; Meng, H. Characterization of critical hemodynamics contributing to aneurysmal remodeling at the basilar terminus in a rabbit model. *Stroke* **2010**, *41*, 1774–1782. [CrossRef] [PubMed]
32. Tutino, V.M.; Mandelbaum, M.; Choi, H.; Pope, L.C.; Siddiqui, A.; Kolega, J.; Meng, H. Aneurysmal remodeling in the circle of Willis after carotid occlusion in an experimental model. *J. Cereb. Blood Flow Metab.* **2014**, *34*, 415–424. [CrossRef] [PubMed]
33. Tutino, V.M.; Mandelbaum, M.; Takahashi, A.; Pope, L.C.; Siddiqui, A.; Kolega, J.; Meng, H. Hypertension and estrogen deficiency augment aneurysmal remodeling in the rabbit circle of willis in response to carotid ligation. *Anat. Rec. (Hoboken)* **2015**, *298*, 1903–1910. [CrossRef]
34. Aoki, T.; Kataoka, H.; Moriwaki, T.; Nozaki, K.; Hashimoto, N. Role of TIMP-1 and TIMP-2 in the progression of cerebral aneurysms. *Stroke* **2007**, *38*, 2337–2345. [CrossRef]
35. Aoki, T.; Fukuda, M.; Nishimura, M.; Nozaki, K.; Narumiya, S. Critical role of TNF-alpha-TNFR1 signaling in intracranial aneurysm formation. *Acta Neuropathol. Commun.* **2014**, *2*, 34. [CrossRef]
36. Coutard, M.; Osborne-Pellegrin, M. Genetic susceptibility to experimental cerebral aneurysm formation in the rat. *Stroke* **1997**, *28*, 1035–1041. [CrossRef]
37. Fukuda, M.; Aoki, T.; Manabe, T.; Maekawa, A.; Shirakawa, T.; Kataoka, H.; Takagi, Y.; Miyamoto, S.; Narumiya, S. Exacerbation of intracranial aneurysm and aortic dissection in hypertensive rat treated with the prostaglandin F-receptor antagonist AS604872. *J. Pharmacol. Sci.* **2014**, *126*, 230–242. [CrossRef]
38. Ikedo, T.; Minami, M.; Kataoka, H.; Hayashi, K.; Nagata, M.; Fujikawa, R.; Higuchi, S.; Yasui, M.; Aoki, T.; Fukuda, M.; et al. Dipeptidyl peptidase-4 inhibitor anagliptin prevents intracranial aneurysm growth by suppressing macrophage infiltration and activation. *J. Am. Heart Assoc.* **2017**, *6*. [CrossRef]
39. Miyata, H.; Koseki, H.; Takizawa, K.; Kasuya, H.; Nozaki, K.; Narumiya, S.; Aoki, T. T cell function is dispensable for intracranial aneurysm formation and progression. *PLoS ONE* **2017**, *12*, e0175421. [CrossRef]
40. Yamamoto, R.; Aoki, T.; Koseki, H.; Fukuda, M.; Hirose, J.; Tsuji, K.; Takizawa, K.; Nakamura, S.; Miyata, H.; Hamakawa, N.; et al. A sphingosine-1-phosphate receptor type 1 agonist, ASP4058, suppresses intracranial aneurysm through promoting endothelial integrity and blocking macrophage transmigration. *Br. J. Pharmacol.* **2017**, *174*, 2085–2101. [CrossRef]
41. Moriwaki, T.; Takagi, Y.; Sadamasa, N.; Aoki, T.; Nozaki, K.; Hashimoto, N. Impaired progression of cerebral aneurysms in interleukin-1beta-deficient mice. *Stroke* **2006**, *37*, 900–905. [CrossRef] [PubMed]
42. Aoki, T.; Kataoka, H.; Morimoto, M.; Nozaki, K.; Hashimoto, N. Macrophage-derived matrix metalloproteinase-2 and -9 promote the progression of cerebral aneurysms in rats. *Stroke* **2007**, *38*, 162–169. [CrossRef] [PubMed]
43. Aoki, T.; Kataoka, H.; Shimamura, M.; Nakagami, H.; Wakayama, K.; Moriwaki, T.; Ishibashi, R.; Nozaki, K.; Morishita, R.; Hashimoto, N. NF-kappaB is a key mediator of cerebral aneurysm formation. *Circulation* **2007**, *116*, 2830–2840. [CrossRef]
44. Aoki, T.; Kataoka, H.; Ishibashi, R.; Nozaki, K.; Hashimoto, N. Simvastatin suppresses the progression of experimentally induced cerebral aneurysms in rats. *Stroke* **2008**, *39*, 1276–1285. [CrossRef]
45. Aoki, T.; Kataoka, H.; Ishibashi, R.; Nozaki, K.; Hashimoto, N. Gene expression profile of the intima and media of experimentally induced cerebral aneurysms in rats by laser-microdissection and microarray techniques. *Int. J. Mol. Med.* **2008**, *22*, 595–603.
46. Aoki, T.; Kataoka, H.; Ishibashi, R.; Nozaki, K.; Hashimoto, N. Cathepsin B, K, and S are expressed in cerebral aneurysms and promote the progression of cerebral aneurysms. *Stroke* **2008**, *39*, 2603–2610. [CrossRef]
47. Aoki, T.; Moriwaki, T.; Takagi, Y.; Kataoka, H.; Yang, J.; Nozaki, K.; Hashimoto, N. The efficacy of apolipoprotein E deficiency in cerebral aneurysm formation. *Int. J. Mol. Med.* **2008**, *21*, 453–459. [CrossRef]
48. Aoki, T.; Kataoka, H.; Ishibashi, R.; Nakagami, H.; Nozaki, K.; Morishita, R.; Hashimoto, N. Pitavastatin suppresses formation and progression of cerebral aneurysms through inhibition of the nuclear factor kappaB pathway. *Neurosurgery* **2009**, *64*, 357–365. [CrossRef]

49. Aoki, T.; Kataoka, H.; Nishimura, M.; Ishibashi, R.; Morishita, R.; Miyamoto, S. Ets-1 promotes the progression of cerebral aneurysm by inducing the expression of MCP-1 in vascular smooth muscle cells. *Gene Ther.* **2010**, *17*, 1117–1123. [CrossRef]
50. Aoki, T.; Nishimura, M.; Ishibashi, R.; Kataoka, H.; Takagi, Y.; Hashimoto, N. Toll-like receptor 4 expression during cerebral aneurysm formation. Laboratory investigation. *J. Neurosurg.* **2010**, *113*, 851–858. [CrossRef]
51. Aoki, T.; Nishimura, M.; Kataoka, H.; Ishibashi, R.; Nozaki, K.; Miyamoto, S. Complementary inhibition of cerebral aneurysm formation by eNOS and nNOS. *Lab. Investig.* **2011**, *91*, 619–626. [CrossRef] [PubMed]
52. Aoki, T.; Kataoka, H.; Nishimura, M.; Ishibashi, R.; Morishita, R.; Miyamoto, S. Regression of intracranial aneurysms by simultaneous inhibition of nuclear factor-kappaB and Ets with chimeric decoy oligodeoxynucleotide treatment. *Neurosurgery* **2012**, *70*, 1534–1543. [CrossRef] [PubMed]
53. Aoki, T.; Frosen, J.; Fukuda, M.; Bando, K.; Shioi, G.; Tsuji, K.; Ollikainen, E.; Nozaki, K.; Laakkonen, J.; Narumiya, S. Prostaglandin E2-EP2-NF-kappaB signaling in macrophages as a potential therapeutic target for intracranial aneurysms. *Sci. Signal.* **2017**, *10*. [CrossRef]
54. Aoki, T.; Saito, M.; Koseki, H.; Tsuji, K.; Tsuji, A.; Murata, K.; Kasuya, H.; Morita, A.; Narumiya, S.; Nozaki, K.; et al. Macrophage imaging of cerebral aneurysms with ferumoxytol: An exploratory study in an animal model and in patients. *J. Stroke Cerebrovasc. Dis.* **2017**, *26*, 2055–2064. [CrossRef] [PubMed]
55. Eldawoody, H.; Shimizu, H.; Kimura, N.; Saito, A.; Nakayama, T.; Takahashi, A.; Tominaga, T. Simplified experimental cerebral aneurysm model in rats: Comprehensive evaluation of induced aneurysms and arterial changes in the circle of Willis. *Brain Res.* **2009**, *1300*, 159–168. [CrossRef]
56. Futami, K.; Yamashita, J.; Tachibana, O.; Higashi, S.; Ikeda, K.; Yamashima, T. Immunohistochemical alterations of fibronectin during the formation and proliferative repair of experimental cerebral aneurysms in rats. *Stroke* **1995**, *26*, 1659–1664. [CrossRef] [PubMed]
57. Futami, K.; Yamashita, J.; Tachibana, O.; Kida, S.; Higashi, S.; Ikeda, K.; Yamashima, T. Basic fibroblast growth factor may repair experimental cerebral aneurysms in rats. *Stroke* **1995**, *26*, 1649–1654. [CrossRef]
58. Futami, K.; Yamashita, J.; Higashi, S. Do cerebral aneurysms originate at the site of medial defects? Microscopic examinations of experimental aneurysms at the fenestration of the anterior cerebral artery in rats. *Surg. Neurol.* **1998**, *50*, 141–146. [CrossRef]
59. Guo, D.; Wang, Y.W.; Ma, J.; Yan, L.; Li, T.F.; Han, X.W.; Shui, S.F. Study on the role of Cathepsin B and JNK signaling pathway in the development of cerebral aneurysm. *Asian Pac. J. Trop. Med.* **2016**, *9*, 499–502. [CrossRef]
60. Hazama, F.; Kataoka, H.; Yamada, E.; Kayembe, K.; Hashimoto, N.; Kojima, M.; Kim, C. Early changes of experimentally induced cerebral aneurysms in rats. Light-microscopic study. *Am. J. Pathol.* **1986**, *124*, 399–404.
61. Ishibashi, R.; Aoki, T.; Nishimura, M.; Hashimoto, N.; Miyamoto, S. Contribution of mast cells to cerebral aneurysm formation. *Curr. Neurovasc. Res.* **2010**, *7*, 113–124. [CrossRef] [PubMed]
62. Jamous, M.A.; Nagahiro, S.; Kitazato, K.T.; Satoh, K.; Satomi, J. Vascular corrosion casts mirroring early morphological changes that lead to the formation of saccular cerebral aneurysm: An experimental study in rats. *J. Neurosurg.* **2005**, *102*, 532–535. [CrossRef] [PubMed]
63. Jamous, M.A.; Nagahiro, S.; Kitazato, K.T.; Satomi, J.; Satoh, K. Role of estrogen deficiency in the formation and progression of cerebral aneurysms. Part I: Experimental study of the effect of oophorectomy in rats. *J. Neurosurg.* **2005**, *103*, 1046–1051. [CrossRef]
64. Jamous, M.A.; Nagahiro, S.; Kitazato, K.T.; Tamura, T.; Kuwayama, K.; Satoh, K. Role of estrogen deficiency in the formation and progression of cerebral aneurysms. Part II: Experimental study of the effects of hormone replacement therapy in rats. *J. Neurosurg.* **2005**, *103*, 1052–1057. [CrossRef]
65. Jamous, M.A.; Nagahiro, S.; Kitazato, K.T.; Tamura, T.; Aziz, H.A.; Shono, M.; Satoh, K. Endothelial injury and inflammatory response induced by hemodynamic changes preceding intracranial aneurysm formation: Experimental study in rats. *J. Neurosurg.* **2007**, *107*, 405–411. [CrossRef]
66. Kang, Y.; Hashimoto, N.; Kikuchi, H.; Yamazoe, N.; Hazama, F. Effects of blood coagulation factor XIII on the development of experimental cerebral aneurysms in rats. *J. Neurosurg.* **1990**, *73*, 242–247. [CrossRef]
67. Kim, C.; Kikuchi, H.; Hashimoto, N.; Kojima, M.; Kang, Y.; Hazama, F. Involvement of internal elastic lamina in development of induced cerebral aneurysms in rats. *Stroke* **1988**, *19*, 507–511. [CrossRef]

68. Kim, C.; Cervos-Navarro, J.; Kikuchi, H.; Hashimoto, N.; Hazama, F. Degenerative changes in the internal elastic lamina relating to the development of saccular cerebral aneurysms in rats. *Acta Neurochir. (Wien)* **1993**, *121*, 76–81. [CrossRef]
69. Kimura, N.; Shimizu, H.; Eldawoody, H.; Nakayama, T.; Saito, A.; Tominaga, T.; Takahashi, A. Effect of olmesartan and pravastatin on experimental cerebral aneurysms in rats. *Brain Res.* **2010**, *1322*, 144–152. [CrossRef]
70. Kojima, M.; Handa, H.; Hashimoto, N.; Kim, C.; Hazama, F. Early changes of experimentally induced cerebral aneurysms in rats: Scanning electron microscopic study. *Stroke* **1986**, *17*, 835–841. [CrossRef]
71. Kondo, S.; Hashimoto, N.; Kikuchi, H.; Hazama, F.; Nagata, I.; Kataoka, H. Cerebral aneurysms arising at nonbranching sites. An experimental Study. *Stroke* **1997**, *28*, 398–403. [CrossRef] [PubMed]
72. Kondo, S.; Hashimoto, N.; Kikuchi, H.; Hazama, F.; Nagata, I.; Kataoka, H. Apoptosis of medial smooth muscle cells in the development of saccular cerebral aneurysms in rats. *Stroke* **1998**, *29*, 181–188. [CrossRef] [PubMed]
73. Korai, M.; Kitazato, K.T.; Tada, Y.; Miyamoto, T.; Shimada, K.; Matsushita, N.; Kanematsu, Y.; Satomi, J.; Hashimoto, T.; Nagahiro, S. Hyperhomocysteinemia induced by excessive methionine intake promotes rupture of cerebral aneurysms in ovariectomized rats. *J. Neuroinflamm.* **2016**, *13*, 165. [CrossRef] [PubMed]
74. Li, S.; Tian, Y.; Huang, X.; Zhang, Y.; Wang, D.; Wei, H.; Dong, J.; Jiang, R.; Zhang, J. Intravenous transfusion of endothelial colony-forming cells attenuates vascular degeneration after cerebral aneurysm induction. *Brain Res.* **2014**, *1593*, 65–75. [CrossRef] [PubMed]
75. Li, S.; Wang, D.; Tian, Y.; Wei, H.; Zhou, Z.; Liu, L.; Wang, D.; Dong, J.F.; Jiang, R.; Zhang, J. Aspirin inhibits degenerative changes of aneurysmal wall in a rat model. *Neurochem. Res.* **2015**, *40*, 1537–1545. [CrossRef]
76. Maekawa, H.; Tada, Y.; Yagi, K.; Miyamoto, T.; Kitazato, K.T.; Korai, M.; Satomi, J.; Hashimoto, T.; Nagahiro, S. Bazedoxifene, a selective estrogen receptor modulator, reduces cerebral aneurysm rupture in Ovariectomized rats. *J. Neuroinflamm.* **2017**, *14*, 197. [CrossRef]
77. Miyamoto, T.; Kung, D.K.; Kitazato, K.T.; Yagi, K.; Shimada, K.; Tada, Y.; Korai, M.; Kurashiki, Y.; Kinouchi, T.; Kanematsu, Y.; et al. Site-specific elevation of interleukin-1beta and matrix metalloproteinase-9 in the Willis circle by hemodynamic changes is associated with rupture in a novel rat cerebral aneurysm model. *J. Cereb. Blood Flow Metab.* **2017**, *37*, 2795–2805. [CrossRef]
78. Nagata, I.; Handa, H.; Hashimoto, N. Experimentally induced cerebral aneurysms in rats: Part IV—Cerebral angiography. *Surg. Neurol.* **1979**, *12*, 419–424.
79. Nagata, I.; Handa, H.; Hashimoto, N.; Hazama, F. Experimentally induced cerebral aneurysms in rats: Part VI. Hypertension. *Surg. Neurol.* **1980**, *14*, 477–479.
80. Nagata, I.; Handa, H.; Hasimoto, N.; Hazama, F. Experimentally induced cerebral aneurysms in rats: VII. Scanning electron microscope study. *Surg. Neurol.* **1981**, *16*, 291–296. [CrossRef]
81. Nakatani, H.; Hashimoto, N.; Kikuchi, H.; Yamaguchi, S.; Niimi, H. In vivo flow visualization of induced saccular cerebral aneurysms in rats. *Acta Neurochir. (Wien)* **1993**, *122*, 244–249. [CrossRef] [PubMed]
82. Sadamasa, N.; Nozaki, K.; Takagi, Y.; Moriwaki, T.; Kawanabe, Y.; Ishikawa, M.; Hashimoto, N. Cerebral aneurysm progression suppressed by blockage of endothelin B receptor. *J. Neurosurg.* **2007**, *106*, 330–336. [CrossRef] [PubMed]
83. Sadamasa, N.; Nozaki, K.; Kita-Matsuo, H.; Saito, S.; Moriwaki, T.; Aoki, T.; Kawarazaki, S.; Kataoka, H.; Takagi, Y.; Ishikawa, M.; et al. Gene expression during the development of experimentally induced cerebral aneurysms. *J. Vasc. Res.* **2008**, *45*, 343–349. [CrossRef] [PubMed]
84. Tada, Y.; Yagi, K.; Kitazato, K.T.; Tamura, T.; Kinouchi, T.; Shimada, K.; Matsushita, N.; Nakajima, N.; Satomi, J.; Kageji, T.; et al. Reduction of endothelial tight junction proteins is related to cerebral aneurysm formation in rats. *J. Hypertens.* **2010**, *28*, 1883–1891. [CrossRef]
85. Tada, Y.; Kitazato, K.T.; Yagi, K.; Shimada, K.; Matsushita, N.; Kinouchi, T.; Kanematsu, Y.; Satomi, J.; Kageji, T.; Nagahiro, S. Statins promote the growth of experimentally induced cerebral aneurysms in estrogen-deficient rats. *Stroke* **2011**, *42*, 2286–2293. [CrossRef]
86. Tamura, T.; Jamous, M.A.; Kitazato, K.T.; Yagi, K.; Tada, Y.; Uno, M.; Nagahiro, S. Endothelial damage due to impaired nitric oxide bioavailability triggers cerebral aneurysm formation in female rats. *J. Hypertens.* **2009**, *27*, 1284–1292. [CrossRef]

87. Yagi, K.; Tada, Y.; Kitazato, K.T.; Tamura, T.; Satomi, J.; Nagahiro, S. Ibudilast inhibits cerebral aneurysms by down-regulating inflammation-related molecules in the vascular wall of rats. *Neurosurgery* **2010**, *66*, 551–559. [CrossRef]
88. Yamazoe, N.; Hashimoto, N.; Kikuchi, H.; Hazama, F. Elastic skeleton of intracranial cerebral aneurysms in rats. *Stroke* **1990**, *21*, 1722–1726. [CrossRef]
89. Yokoi, T.; Isono, T.; Saitoh, M.; Yoshimura, Y.; Nozaki, K. Suppression of cerebral aneurysm formation in rats by a tumor necrosis factor-alpha inhibitor. *J. Neurosurg.* **2014**, *120*, 1193–1200. [CrossRef]
90. Wu, C.; Liu, Y.; He, M.; Zhu, L.; You, C. Single operation with simplified incisions to build an experimental cerebral aneurysm model by induced hemodynamic stress and estrogen deficiency in rats. *Turk. Neurosurg.* **2016**, *26*, 62–68. [CrossRef]
91. Zhou, D.; Bao, Y.D.; Du, Z.W.; Takeda, F.; Kanno, T. Experimental cerebral aneurysms in rats. Experimental method and effect of estradiol. *Chin. Med. J. (Engl.)* **1985**, *98*, 421–426. [PubMed]
92. Sadamasa, N.; Nozaki, K.; Hashimoto, N. Disruption of gene for inducible nitric oxide synthase reduces progression of cerebral aneurysms. *Stroke* **2003**, *34*, 2980–2984. [CrossRef] [PubMed]
93. Zhao, J.; Lin, X.; He, C.; Yang, G.Y.; Ling, F. Study of cerebral aneurysms in a modified rat model: From real-time imaging to histological analysis. *J. Clin. Neurosci.* **2015**, *22*, 373–377. [CrossRef] [PubMed]
94. Chalouhi, N.; Starke, R.M.; Correa, T.; Jabbour, P.M.; Zanaty, M.; Brown, R.D., Jr.; Torner, J.C.; Hasan, D.M. Differential sex response to aspirin in decreasing aneurysm rupture in humans and mice. *Hypertension* **2016**, *68*, 411–417. [CrossRef]
95. Chu, Y.; Wilson, K.; Gu, H.; Wegman-Points, L.; Dooley, S.A.; Pierce, G.L.; Cheng, G.; Pena Silva, R.A.; Heistad, D.D.; Hasan, D. Myeloperoxidase is increased in human cerebral aneurysms and increases formation and rupture of cerebral aneurysms in mice. *Stroke* **2015**, *46*, 1651–1656. [CrossRef]
96. Hasan, D.M.; Starke, R.M.; Gu, H.; Wilson, K.; Chu, Y.; Chalouhi, N.; Heistad, D.D.; Faraci, F.M.; Sigmund, C.D. Smooth muscle peroxisome proliferator-activated receptor gamma plays a critical role in formation and rupture of cerebral aneurysms in mice in vivo. *Hypertension* **2015**, *66*, 211–220. [CrossRef]
97. Kanematsu, Y.; Kanematsu, M.; Kurihara, C.; Tada, Y.; Tsou, T.L.; van Rooijen, N.; Lawton, M.T.; Young, W.L.; Liang, E.I.; Nuki, Y.; et al. Critical roles of macrophages in the formation of intracranial aneurysm. *Stroke* **2011**, *42*, 173–178. [CrossRef]
98. Kuwabara, A.; Liu, J.; Kamio, Y.; Liu, A.; Lawton, M.T.; Lee, J.W.; Hashimoto, T. Protective effect of mesenchymal stem cells against the development of intracranial aneurysm rupture in mice. *Neurosurgery* **2017**, *81*, 1021–1028. [CrossRef]
99. Labeyrie, P.E.; Goulay, R.; Martinez de Lizarrondo, S.; Hebert, M.; Gauberti, M.; Maubert, E.; Delaunay, B.; Gory, B.; Signorelli, F.; Turjman, F.; et al. Vascular tissue-type plasminogen activator promotes intracranial aneurysm formation. *Stroke* **2017**, *48*, 2574–2582. [CrossRef]
100. Lee, J.A.; Marshman, L.A.; Moran, C.S.; Kuma, L.; Guazzo, E.P.; Anderson, D.S.; Golledge, J. A small animal model for early cerebral aneurysm pathology. *J. Clin. Neurosci.* **2016**, *34*, 259–263. [CrossRef]
101. Liu, J.; Kuwabara, A.; Kamio, Y.; Hu, S.; Park, J.; Hashimoto, T.; Lee, J.W. Human mesenchymal stem cell-derived microvesicles prevent the rupture of intracranial aneurysm in part by suppression of mast cell activation via a pge2-dependent mechanism. *Stem Cells* **2016**, *34*, 2943–2955. [CrossRef] [PubMed]
102. Liu, M.; Zhao, J.; Zhou, Q.; Peng, Y.; Zhou, Y.; Jiang, Y. Primary cilia deficiency induces intracranial aneurysm. *Shock* **2018**, *49*, 604–611. [CrossRef] [PubMed]
103. Makino, H.; Tada, Y.; Wada, K.; Liang, E.I.; Chang, M.; Mobashery, S.; Kanematsu, Y.; Kurihara, C.; Palova, E.; Kanematsu, M.; et al. Pharmacological stabilization of intracranial aneurysms in mice: A feasibility study. *Stroke* **2012**, *43*, 2450–2456. [CrossRef]
104. Makino, H.; Hokamura, K.; Natsume, T.; Kimura, T.; Kamio, Y.; Magata, Y.; Namba, H.; Katoh, T.; Sato, S.; Hashimoto, T.; et al. Successful serial imaging of the mouse cerebral arteries using conventional 3-T magnetic resonance imaging. *J. Cereb. Blood Flow Metab.* **2015**, *35*, 1523–1527. [CrossRef]
105. Nuki, Y.; Tsou, T.L.; Kurihara, C.; Kanematsu, M.; Kanematsu, Y.; Hashimoto, T. Elastase-induced intracranial aneurysms in hypertensive mice. *Hypertension* **2009**, *54*, 1337–1344. [CrossRef] [PubMed]
106. Pena Silva, R.A.; Kung, D.K.; Mitchell, I.J.; Alenina, N.; Bader, M.; Santos, R.A.; Faraci, F.M.; Heistad, D.D.; Hasan, D.M. Angiotensin 1–7 reduces mortality and rupture of intracranial aneurysms in mice. *Hypertension* **2014**, *64*, 362–368. [CrossRef] [PubMed]

107. Pena-Silva, R.A.; Chalouhi, N.; Wegman-Points, L.; Ali, M.; Mitchell, I.; Pierce, G.L.; Chu, Y.; Ballas, Z.K.; Heistad, D.; Hasan, D. Novel role for endogenous hepatocyte growth factor in the pathogenesis of intracranial aneurysms. *Hypertension* **2015**, *65*, 587–593. [CrossRef]
108. Shimada, K.; Furukawa, H.; Wada, K.; Korai, M.; Wei, Y.; Tada, Y.; Kuwabara, A.; Shikata, F.; Kitazato, K.T.; Nagahiro, S.; et al. Protective role of peroxisome proliferator-activated receptor-gamma in the development of intracranial aneurysm rupture. *Stroke* **2015**, *46*, 1664–1672. [CrossRef]
109. Shimada, K.; Furukawa, H.; Wada, K.; Wei, Y.; Tada, Y.; Kuwabara, A.; Shikata, F.; Kanematsu, Y.; Lawton, M.T.; Kitazato, K.T.; et al. Angiotensin-(1-7) protects against the development of aneurysmal subarachnoid hemorrhage in mice. *J. Cereb. Blood Flow Metab.* **2015**, *35*, 1163–1168. [CrossRef]
110. Tada, Y.; Makino, H.; Furukawa, H.; Shimada, K.; Wada, K.; Liang, E.I.; Murakami, S.; Kudo, M.; Kung, D.K.; Hasan, D.M.; et al. Roles of estrogen in the formation of intracranial aneurysms in ovariectomized female mice. *Neurosurgery* **2014**, *75*, 690–695. [CrossRef]
111. Tada, Y.; Wada, K.; Shimada, K.; Makino, H.; Liang, E.I.; Murakami, S.; Kudo, M.; Kitazato, K.T.; Nagahiro, S.; Hashimoto, T. Roles of hypertension in the rupture of intracranial aneurysms. *Stroke* **2014**, *45*, 579–586. [CrossRef] [PubMed]
112. Tada, Y.; Wada, K.; Shimada, K.; Makino, H.; Liang, E.I.; Murakami, S.; Kudo, M.; Shikata, F.; Pena Silva, R.A.; Kitazato, K.T.; et al. Estrogen protects against intracranial aneurysm rupture in ovariectomized mice. *Hypertension* **2014**, *63*, 1339–1344. [CrossRef]
113. Wada, K.; Makino, H.; Shimada, K.; Shikata, F.; Kuwabara, A.; Hashimoto, T. Translational research using a mouse model of intracranial aneurysm. *Transl. Stroke Res.* **2014**, *5*, 248–251. [CrossRef]
114. Zhang, M.; Ren, Y.; Wang, Y.; Wang, R.; Zhou, Q.; Peng, Y.; Li, Q.; Yu, M.; Jiang, Y. Regulation of smooth muscle contractility by competing endogenous mRNAs in intracranial aneurysms. *J. Neuropathol. Exp. Neurol.* **2015**, *74*, 411–424. [CrossRef]
115. Dai, D.; Ding, Y.H.; Kadirvel, R.; Lewis, D.A.; Kallmes, D.F. Experience with microaneurysm formation at the basilar terminus in the rabbit elastase aneurysm model. *AJNR Am. J. Neuroradiol.* **2010**, *31*, 300–303. [CrossRef]
116. Yasuda, H.; Kuroda, S.; Nanba, R.; Ishikawa, T.; Shinya, N.; Terasaka, S.; Iwasaki, Y.; Nagashima, K. A novel coating biomaterial for intracranial aneurysms: Effects and safety in extra- and intracranial carotid artery. *Neuropathology* **2005**, *25*, 66–76. [CrossRef]
117. Hoh, B.L.; Hosaka, K.; Downes, D.P.; Nowicki, K.W.; Wilmer, E.N.; Velat, G.J.; Scott, E.W. Stromal cell-derived factor-1 promoted angiogenesis and inflammatory cell infiltration in aneurysm walls. *J. Neurosurg.* **2014**, *120*, 73–86. [CrossRef]
118. Hosaka, K.; Downes, D.P.; Nowicki, K.W.; Hoh, B.L. Modified murine intracranial aneurysm model: Aneurysm formation and rupture by elastase and hypertension. *J. Neurointerv. Surg.* **2014**, *6*, 474–479. [CrossRef]
119. Hosaka, K.; Rojas, K.; Fazal, H.Z.; Schneider, M.B.; Shores, J.; Federico, V.; McCord, M.; Lin, L.; Hoh, B. Monocyte chemotactic protein-1-interleukin-6-osteopontin pathway of intra-aneurysmal tissue healing. *Stroke* **2017**, *48*, 1052–1060. [CrossRef]
120. Nowicki, K.W.; Hosaka, K.; Walch, F.J.; Scott, E.W.; Hoh, B.L. M1 macrophages are required for murine cerebral aneurysm formation. *J. Neurointerv. Surg.* **2018**, *10*, 93–97. [CrossRef]
121. Lee, J.; Berry, C.L. Cerebral micro-aneurysm formation in the hypertensive rat. *J. Pathol.* **1978**, *124*, 7–11. [CrossRef] [PubMed]
122. Tada, Y.; Kitazato, K.T.; Tamura, T.; Yagi, K.; Shimada, K.; Kinouchi, T.; Satomi, J.; Nagahiro, S. Role of mineralocorticoid receptor on experimental cerebral aneurysms in rats. *Hypertension* **2009**, *54*, 552–557. [CrossRef] [PubMed]
123. Jung, K.H.; Chu, K.; Lee, S.T.; Shin, Y.W.; Lee, K.J.; Park, D.K.; Yoo, J.S.; Kim, S.; Kim, M.; Lee, S.K.; et al. Experimental induction of cerebral aneurysms by developmental low copper diet. *J. Neuropathol. Exp. Neurol.* **2016**, *75*, 455–463. [CrossRef] [PubMed]
124. Bo, L.J.; Miao, Z.; Wang, Z.F.; Zhang, K.Z.; Gao, Z. A study on effect of curcumin on anticerebral aneurysm in the male albino rats. *Brain Behav.* **2017**, *7*, e00729. [CrossRef]
125. Ebina, K.; Iwabuchi, T.; Suzuki, S. A clinico-experimental study on various wrapping materials of cerebral aneurysms. *Acta Neurochir. (Wien)* **1984**, *72*, 61–71. [CrossRef]

126. Nishikawa, M.; Smith, R.D.; Yonekawa, Y. Experimental intracranial aneurysms. *Surg. Neurol.* **1977**, *7*, 241–244.
127. Gopal, K.; Nagarajan, P.; Raj, T.A.; Jahan, P.; Ganapathy, H.S.; Mahesh Kumar, M.J. Effect of dietary beta carotene on cerebral aneurysm and subarachnoid haemorrhage in the brain apo E−/− mice. *J. Thromb. Thrombolysis* **2011**, *32*, 343–355. [CrossRef]
128. CAMARADES. Collaborative Approach to Meta-Analysis and Review of Animal Data from Experimental Studies. Available online: http://www.dcn.ed.ac.uk/camarades/ (accessed on 1 August 2019).

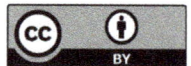

© 2020 by the authors. Licensee MDPI, Basel, Switzerland. This article is an open access article distributed under the terms and conditions of the Creative Commons Attribution (CC BY) license (http://creativecommons.org/licenses/by/4.0/).

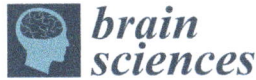

Review

Saccular Aneurysm Models Featuring Growth and Rupture: A Systematic Review

Serge Marbacher [1,2,*], Stefan Wanderer [1,2], Fabio Strange [1,2], Basil E. Grüter [1,2] and Javier Fandino [1,2]

1. Department of Neurosurgery, Kantonsspital Aarau, Aarau 5000, Switzerland; stefan.wanderer@ksa.ch (S.W.); fabio.strange@ksa.ch (F.S.); basil.grueter@ksa.ch (B.E.G.); javier.fandino@ksa.ch (J.F.)
2. Cerebrovascular Research Group, Department for BioMedical Research, University of Bern, Bern 3000, Switzerland
* Correspondence: serge.marbacher@ksa.ch; Tel.: +41-62-838-5970

Received: 15 January 2020; Accepted: 25 January 2020; Published: 13 February 2020

Abstract: Background. Most available large animal extracranial aneurysm models feature healthy non-degenerated aneurysm pouches with stable long-term follow-ups and extensive healing reactions after endovascular treatment. This review focuses on a small subgroup of extracranial aneurysm models that demonstrated growth and potential rupture during follow-up. Methods. The literature was searched in Medline/Pubmed to identify extracranial in vivo saccular aneurysm models featuring growth and rupture, using a predefined search strategy in accordance with the PRISMA guidelines. From eligible studies we extracted the following details: technique and location of aneurysm creation, aneurysm pouch characteristics, time for model creation, growth and rupture rate, time course, patency rate, histological findings, and associated morbidity and mortality. Results. A total of 20 articles were found to describe growth and/or rupture of an experimentally created extracranial saccular aneurysm during follow-up. Most frequent growth was reported in rats ($n = 6$), followed by rabbits ($n = 4$), dogs ($n = 4$), swine ($n = 5$), and sheep ($n = 1$). Except for two studies reporting growth and rupture within the abdominal cavity (abdominal aortic artery; $n = 2$) all other aneurysms were located at the neck of the animal. The largest growth rate, with an up to 10-fold size increase, was found in a rat abdominal aortic sidewall aneurysm model. Conclusions. Extracranial saccular aneurysm models with growth and rupture are rare. Degradation of the created aneurysmal outpouch seems to be a prerequisite to allow growth, which may ultimately lead to rupture. Since it has been shown that the aneurysm wall is important for healing after endovascular therapy, it is likely that models featuring growth and rupture will gain in interest for preclinical testing of novel endovascular therapies.

Keywords: animal model; growth; aneurysm rupture; saccular; intracranial aneurysm

1. Introduction

Increased understanding of the complex pathobiology of intracranial aneurysm (IA) growth, rupture, and the effects of endovascular therapy depends on epidemiological data analysis, clinical findings, histopathology of IA samples obtained during surgery, and gene linkage analysis [1–5] Experimental work using animal models of IA are needed to delineate the biological mechanisms of IA formation and growth, and to establish new medical and endovascular therapies and materials to prevent IA rupture. Cerebral aneurysm models can be divided into two large groups: Intra- and extracranial models [6].

There is a growing body of evidence that the aneurysm wall condition influences the healing response and long-term durability after endovascular therapy [7–10]. Most available extracranial aneurysm models feature healthy non-degenerated aneurysm pouches with stable long-term follow-ups and extensive healing reactions after endovascular treatment [11]. This review focuses on a small subgroup of extracranial saccular aneurysm models that demonstrate growth and potential rupture during follow-up. It is likely that this subgroup of models will become more important for challenging the testing of devices prior to their clinical application [6,7,12]. This systematic review provides a comprehensive overview of available techniques and associated characteristics of extracranial aneurysm models featuring growth and rupture. Furthermore, this summary serves as reference for the development of novel models and supports researchers in the planning and execution of their future experiments.

2. Materials and Methods

2.1. Literature Search

The literature was searched in Medline/Pubmed on November 31, 2017 to identify extracranial in vivo saccular aneurysm models featuring growth and rupture using a predefined search strategy. Briefly, we used the following key words: "murine", "rat", "rabbit", "canine", "primate", "cat", "pig", "sheep", and "goat" in combination with "intracranial aneurysm" using the Boolean operator [AND]. The search was restricted to animals and two investigators (SM and FS) independently screened titles and abstracts for eligible studies and removed duplicates. Full text analysis of the remaining articles determined their final eligibility. Uncertainties by the two investigators were discussed with a third examiner (BG). Cross-references were searched until no further studies were identified. The search algorithm was in accordance with the PRISMA guidelines.

2.2. Eligibility Criteria and Analyzed Features

We considered all preclinical extracranial saccular aneurysm models with documented growth and/or rupture. We excluded in vitro experiments, studies on intracranial vessels, studies published in a language other than English, articles designed for the study of thoracic or abdominal aortic aneurysms, and review articles. From each study included in the final analysis we recorded the following: authors, year of publication, aneurysm model category (sidewall, terminal, stump, bifurcation, and complex), species, detailed technique of aneurysm creation, aneurysm pouch characteristics (vital or modified, arterial or venous), initial size and location of the aneurysms, time for model creation, growth rate and time course of growth, size of increase (as percentage of baseline), rupture rate and time course, patency rate, mortality and morbidity rate, and histological findings.

3. Results

A total of 20 articles were found that described growth and/or rupture of an experimentally created extracranial saccular aneurysm. The initial electronic search yielded 4264 potential studies. Of these, 3788 articles were excluded after title and abstract screening and 4 articles were excluded after identification of duplicates. The remaining 472 articles underwent full text analysis. Of those, 405 studies were excluded according to the predefined eligibility criteria. Another 48 studies describing various saccular aneurysm models were excluded because none of the reported techniques resulted in growth or rupture of the created aneurysms. One study was added by cross-referencing (Figure 1).

Growth and/or rupture of experimental aneurysms were found in three types of models: sidewall (n = 12) [3,8,13–22], bifurcation stump (n = 6) [14,23–27], and terminal (n = 3) [28–30]. Most frequent growth was reported in rats (n = 6) [8,14,16,23–25], followed by rabbits (n = 4) [13,21,26,29], dogs (n = 4) [19,27,28,30], swine (n = 5) [3,17,18,20,22], and sheep (n = 1) [15]. Except for two studies reporting growth and rupture within the abdominal cavity (abdominal aortic artery; n = 2) [8,16] all other aneurysms were located at the neck of the animal (common carotid artery; n = 18). The identified 20 models used in n = 14 venous pouches (in n = 2 of them inverted venous pouches [3,30]), in n = 3 modified arterial pouches (n = 2 porcine elastase [26,29] and n = 1 sodium dodecyl sulfate [8]), and in n = 3 direct mechanical arterial wall weakening [13,23,24] to create growing and rupture-prone aneurysms. Time for aneurysm creation was reported in only two studies (180 minutes each for a terminal model in dogs [28] and rabbits [29]).

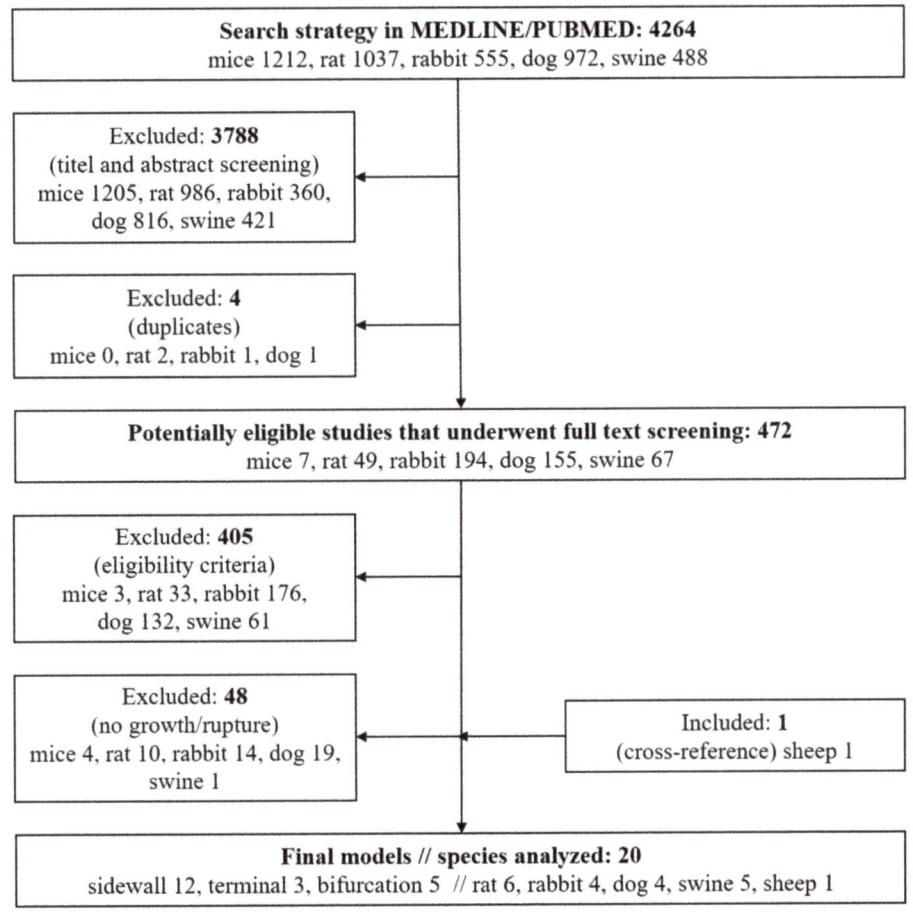

Figure 1. PRISMA flow chart for study selection.

Almost half (*n* = 9 out of 20) of the models demonstrated growth only without associated rupture during follow-up. The volume increase varied greatly between the models used and ranged between tiny blebs [23] and a 10-fold increase [8] in initial size. Most models (*n* = 17 out of 20) reported only modest increase, with stabilization at further follow-up. The largest increase in aneurysm volume was found in rat sidewall aneurysm models created in the abdominal cavity. Growth rate and time course of growth ranged from 23% to 100% and from weeks to months, respectively.

More than half (*n* = 11 out of 20) of all identified models reported rupture during follow-up. In three out of these eleven models the aneurysm wall was modified at the time of creation [8,26,29]. Intraluminal aneurysm thrombosis was present in 9 out of 11 models featuring rupture. Rupture occurred within a few days and up to months after aneurysm creation. Except for a single case of rupture within one day all other ruptures occurred later than day 3 after creation, irrespective of the model applied. The rate of rupture ranged from 7% to 100% depending on the model used. Associated morbidity and mortality ranged from 0% to 50%. Three studies did not report associated morbidity and mortality rate.

Table 1. Detailed characteristics of aneurysm models featuring growth and rupture.

#	Author (Year)	Animal	Location // Size (Baseline)	Model (Pouch) // Time for Creation	Modified Wall // Thrombus	Growth Rate and Time Course // Patency Rate // Size Increase from Baseline (%)	Rupture Rate and Time Course // Mortality and Morbidity	Histological Findings
1	Troupp and Rinne (1964) [13]	Rabbit	Rt CCA // NR	Sidewall // NR	Yes (arteriotomy glued with Methyl-2-Cyanoacrylate) // NR	32% (16/50) within 4–21 weeks // 38% (6/16) within 4–13 weeks // NR	None // 6% (3/50) mortality	NR
2	Nishikawa et al. (1976) [14]	Rat	CCA // 2.15 ± 0.39 mm (length) × 1.55 ± 0.34 mm (width) × 0.88 ± 0.36 mm (height)	Sidewall and true bifurcation (venous pouch, AFV) // NR	No // 4% (4/112)	Growth within the first week // 96% (108/112) // 24% (length), 25% (width) and 42% (height)	8% (9/112) rupture in both models (sidewall and true bifurcation) // 4.46% (5/112)	Thickening of the aneurysm wall, when the aneurysm had existed for a long time
3	Stehbens (1979) [15]	Sheep	CCA // NR	Sidewall (venous pouch, EJV) // NR	No // 41% (11/27)	No notable growth // NR // NR	30% (8/27) within 3 weeks // 30% (8/27) within 3 weeks	Detailed description of histological changes in the aneurysm sac and parent artery. All ruptured aneurysms contained macroscopic thrombus
4	Young et al. (1987) [23]	Rat	CCA // 2 × 2 mm	True bifurcation // NR	Yes (external mural excision) // NR	Aneurysms grew into tiny blebs of various shape and sizes at 3–12 weeks FU // NR // NR	55.5% (5/9) // NR	Aneurysms were usually small and broad-based with noticeably thin walls
5	Gao et al. (1990) [24]	Rat	CCA // 0.8 ± 0.3 mm (length) × 0.7 ± 0.2 mm (width) ± 0.4 ± 0.1 mm (height)	True bifurcation // NR	Yes (transluminal removal of the tunica intima and media) // 0% (0/20)	Significant growth of all 20/20 aneurysm within the first 2 months remained stable until 3 months FU // 70% (14/20) after 2 months, 60% (6/10) after 3 month // 37.5% length, 28.57% width, 50% height	0% (0/20) // 0% (0/20)	No thrombosis, endothelial cells covered smooth surface. IEL and tunica media absent; regenerative elastic fibers. Disorderly arranged fibroblast-like without pattern and dispersive. Vasa vasorum and few foam cells occasionally in the experimental wall between the collagenous and elastic fibers. Tunica adventitia intact and infiltrated by some mononuclear cells and foreign body giant cells
6	Sadasivan et al. (1990) [16]	Rat	AA // 3 mm	Sidewall (venous pouch, IJV) // NR	No // 6.45% (4/62)	Growth occurred after wrapping with cotton or polyvinyl alcohol // 100% (62/62) // NR	NR // NR	All giant aneurysms (n = 4) were partially thrombosed. Two in each wrapping group
7	Graves et al. (1993) [28]	Dog	Both CCA // 15 mm (width), 21 mm (height)	Terminal (venous pouch, EJV) // 180 min	No // NR	Increase in size over time at 13 weeks (9–17 weeks) // 100% (6/6) // average increase 33% width, 9.52% height	0% (0/6) // 0% (0/6)	NR
8	Byrne et al. (1994) [17]	Swine	CCA // 15–20 mm (length)	Sidewall (venous pouch, EJV) embolized with GDC // NR	No // 14.28% (1/7)	Tendency for growth in aneurysms with partial thrombosis // 14.28 (1/7) after 2–3 weeks // NR	100% (4/4) of untreated aneurysm within 4 ± 0.5 days; 75% (3/4) of partial (<90%) occlusion using GDC within 4 ± 1 days // 50% (7/14)	Marked edema and acute inflammatory infiltration of the whole wall, wall dissection, and necrosis of smooth muscle fibers
9	Kirse et al. (1996) [25]	Rat	Both CCA // 1.40 mm (width) × 3.125 mm (height)	Artificial bifurcation (venous pouch, EJV) // NR	No // 33.33% (4/12)	1.45 mm (width), 3.45 mm (height) after 1 week, 2.4 mm (width), 3.875 mm (height) after 3 weeks, 2.1 mm (width), 4.175 mm (height) after 3 months // 100% (12/12) // Average volume increases 21.5% after 1 week, 96% after 3 weeks and 145% within 3 months	NR // NR	Small adventitial collections of lymphocytes, some pigment-laden macrophages, and focal foreign body giant cell reaction to suture material. The endothelial surfaces were intact and continuous and the lumens patent
10	Raymond et al. (1999) [18]	Swine	CCA // NR	Sidewall (venous pouch, EJV) embolized with collagen sponges 95% (25/30) or Guglielmi Detachable coils 5% (5/30) // NR	No // NR	NR // 100% (25/25) // NR	80% (4/5) rupture of residual aneurysm after embolization within 3–5 days // 16% (5/30) mortality	Healing responses following embolization of porcine aneurysms with GDC or Gelfoam sponges were essentially similar at 3 weeks

Table 1. *Cont.*

#	Author (Year)	Animal	Location // Size (Baseline)	Model (Pouch) // Time for Creation	Modified Wall // Thrombus	Growth Rate and Time Course // Patency Rate // Size Increase from Baseline (%)	Rupture Rate and Time Course // Mortality and Morbidity	Histological Findings
11	Fujiwara et al. (2001) [26]	Rabbit	CCA // NR	Bifurcation stump // NR	Yes (arterial pouch, CCA modified with porcine elastase (Sigma, St. Louis) for 20 min in 66.66% (6/9)) // NR	100% growth rate (6/6) within 1 month (day 3.3.2 ± 0.6 mm (width), 6.0 ± 1.3 mm (height); day 14 4.1 ± 1.7 mm (width), 8.3 ± 1.9 mm (height); 35 days 5.0 ± 0.9 mm (width), 10.0 ± 2.2 mm (height) with stable course up to 4 months in the elastase group // 100% (9/9) // NR	0% (0/9) // 0% (0/9)	NR (control animals without elastase infusion did not show dilation of the stump at any timepoint (3–21 days) after aneurysm creation)
12	Yang et al. (2001) [14]	Dog	CCA // 6–8 mm (diameter), 3–4 mm (neck)	Sidewall (venous pouch, EJV) embolized with CAP // NR	No // 84.61% (11/13) with CAP treatment	16.66% (1/6) of partially thrombosed aneurysm enlarged between 4–8 weeks // 25% (3/12) // NR	33.33% (2/6) of total and subtotal occluded aneurysms ruptured at day 4 and 5 // 33.33% (2/6)	Endothelial cells and basal membrane were destroyed. Fibrous cells and SMC showed obvious degeneration. Inflammatory cells most prominent 1–2 weeks after thrombosis
13	Murayama et al. (2003) [22]	Swine	CCA // 8–12 mm (diameter), 7 mm (neck)	Sidewall (venous pouch, EJV) embolized with GDC or Matrix // NR	No // GDC 100% (23/23) and 100% (26/26) after 6 months	NR // NR // 14.6% from baseline to day 14 in the GDC group, 19.68% vs. baseline in the Matrix group; 4.09% from baseline to day 14 for the GDC group after 3 months, 6 months NA for the GDC- and Matrix group	23% (3/13): 5 days (2/13) and 12 days (1/13) after GDC embolization // 11.5% (3/26)	Unorganized intraluminal clot (5 day) and large neck hematoma (day 12), rupture point at the dome of the venous pouch
14	Becker et al. (2007) [33]	Swine	CCA // 8.9 mm (height), 8.2 mm (width), 7.7 mm (depth)	Sidewall (venous pouch, EJV) embolized with calcium alginate // NR	No // 100% (8/8)	NR // 0% (0/8) in treatment group within 3 months, 100% (2/2) in control group of partial occlusion (<50%) within 8 days // NR	100% (2/2) of partial occlusion (<50%) after 6 and 8 days // 20% (2/10)	Inflammatory cell infiltration in aneurysm sac and neutrophil infiltration within unorganized thrombus
15	Yang et al. (2007) [29]	Rabbit	Both CCA // 8 mm (length)	Terminal // 180 min	Yes (arterial pouch, CCA modified with Hanks solution containing elastase (60 U/ml) for 20 min and collagenase typ I for 15 min) // 33.33% (3/9)	100% (9/9) within 1–2 weeks // NR // mean diameter increased 60% after 2 weeks (from 2.0 ± 0.1 mm to 3.2 ± 0.3 mm)	33.33% (3/9), one each after 1 day, 2 weeks, and 4 weeks // 40% (4/10)	Differentiation of tunica intima, media and adventitia was lost. Fragmentation of elastic laminar. Thinning of the wall composed of a thin layer of acellular fibrous tissue/collagen
16	Tsumoto et al. (2008) [27]	Dog	Both CCA // NR	Artificial bifurcation (venous pouch, EJV) // NR	No // 20% (1/5)	100% (5/5) within 10 months FU // 80% (4/5) // Significant increase after 10 months 18.7 ± 1.3 mm (height), 11.1 ± 1.9 mm (width), 8.1 ± 1.4 mm (neck)	0% (0/5) // 0% (0/5)	Aneurysms increase in size (height, width, and neck diameter) during the 1–4 months over a 10-month period. No significant differences in dimensions between 7 and 10 months
17	Naggara et al. (2010) [30]	Dog	Both CCA and IT // 13.9 ± 3.3 mm (fundus), 3.6 ± 1.2 mm (neck)	Terminal // NR	Yes (venous pouch, EJV, inverted) // NR	100% (16/16) within 1 month, then remained stable up to 10 months // 100% (16/16) at 9.0 ± 3.6 months FU // 19.19% fundus increase after up to 10 months (from 13.9 to 17.2 mm), 26.54% neck increase after up to 10 months (from 3.6 to 4.9 mm)	0% (0/16) // 0% (0/16)	NR
18	Ding et al. (2012) [21]	Rabbit	CCA // 2.4 ± 0.4 mm (neck), 4.3 ± 1.2 mm (width), 4.3 ± 1.4 mm (height)	Sidewall (venous pouch, EJV) // NR	No // NR	95% (38/40) increase within 3 weeks // 95% (38/40) aneurysms remained patent // 150% increase after 3 weeks (from 51 mm³ to 127.5 mm³)	0% (0/40) // 0% (0/40)	However, no data whether further growth occurred later than 1 month after creation

Table 1. Cont.

#	Author (Year)	Animal	Location // Size (Baseline)	Model (Pouch) // Time for Creation	Modified Wall // Thrombus	Growth Rate and Time Course // Patency Rate // Size Increase from Baseline (%)	Rupture Rate and Time Course // Mortality and Morbidity	Histological Findings
19	Raymond et al. (2012) [3]	Swine	Both CCA // group 1: 11.3 ± 2.6 mm (long axis), 6.7 ± 2.1 mm (short axis); group 2: 5.8 ± 0.6 mm (neck); 16.9 mm ± 4.0 mm (long axis), 8.1 mm ± 1.3 mm (short axis), 4.8 mm ± 1.1 mm (neck); group 3 26.1 ± 10.09 mm (long axis), 9.4 ± 1.4 mm (short axis), 5.8 ± 1.0 mm (neck)	Sidewall // NR	Yes (venous pouch, EJV, removal of endothelial lining) // 83.33% (20/24)	NR // 54.16% (26/48): group 1 remained patent at 2 weeks, partially occluded at 3 weeks, completely occluded in 4 weeks (n = 12); group 2 fully occluded at 2 weeks in 2 animals without rupture (n = 8); group 3 lesions clipped were confirmed to be completely occluded immediately postoperatively and at 7 days (n=6) // NR	50% (2/4) of small size with small neck in group 2 within 2 weeks, 100% (7/7) of giant size with wide neck in group 3 (untreated) within 1 weeks, 16.66% (1/6) of giant size with wide neck in group 3 (clipped); in total 41.66% (10/24) // 20.83% (5/24)	Intraluminal unorganized thrombus in all ruptured aneurysm, many areas with loss of SMC and elastic fibers, inflammatory cells infiltrating the venous wall, hemorrhagic wall transformation
20	Marbacher et al. (2014) [5]	Rat	AA // 2.5 ± 0.3 mm (width) control group, 2.6 ± 0.2 (width) SDS group; 4.2 ± 0.4 mm (length) control group, 4.1 ± 0.6 mm (length) control group	Sidewall // NR	Yes (arterial pouch, syngeneic TA modified with SDS 0.1% for 6 hours to decellularize the wall) // 13% (3/10) in the control group after 4 weeks, 33% (2/6) in the SDS group after 4 weeks	33% (4/12) within 1 week, largest growth (43 × 38 × 24 mm) with 10x increase in size // 38% (3/8) in the control group after 4 weeks, 50% (3/6) in the SDS group after 4 weeks // up to 1000%	75% (3/4) earliest rupture within eleven days after creation // 18.75% (3/16)	Unorganized intraluminal thrombus, strong adventitial and wall inflammation, marked inflammatory cells in medial matrix, luminal thrombus with neutrophils. Wall dissection and mural hematomas. Loss of EC and SMC

Rt = Right; Lt = Left; NR = not reported; CCA = common carotid artery; AFV = anterior facial vein; EJV = external jugular vein; IJV = internal jugular vein; FU = follow-up; IEL = internal elastic lamina; AA = abdominal aorta; IJV = internal jugular vein; GDC = Guglielmi detachable coil; CAP = cellulose acetate polymer; SMC = smooth muscle cell; EC = endothelial cell; IT = innominate trunk; TA = thoracic aorta; SDS = sodium dodecyl sulfate.

The predominant histological findings in growing and ruptured aneurysms are: unorganized intraluminal thrombus, incomplete neointima formation with partial aneurysm recurrence, marked inflammatory cells within unorganized thrombus and aneurysm wall, hemorrhagic transformation of the aneurysm wall with intramural loss of endothelial cells, smooth muscle cells, and degradation of extracellular matrix components. All details of each model and associated characteristics are summarized in Table 1.

4. Discussion

Most extracranial aneurysm models differ from human saccular aneurysms not only in their histology, but their reluctance towards growth and rupture. In consequence, aneurysm growth and/or rupture during follow-up are rare events. This review demonstrates that the following characteristics seem to be associated with growth and rupture of extracranial saccular aneurysms, regardless of the species or model used: intraluminal aneurysm thrombosis, intraluminal and intramural inflammation, endothelial and mural cell loss, and hemorrhagic transformation of the aneurysm wall. Most of the identified 20 extracranial saccular aneurysm models were of sidewall type and featured only short-term aneurysm maturation rather than true aneurysm growth during follow-up.

After pioneering work on aneurysm creation by direct vessel manipulation on extra- and intracranial arteries by McCune et al. [31] and White et al. [32] it was Troupp and Rinne [13] who demonstrated the growth of sidewall carotid aneurysms in rabbits created by an arteriotomy glued with methl-2-cyanoacrylate. They found significant increase in size in 30% of aneurysms over a time of 1 to 5 months. Many models demonstrate maturation by means of aneurysm enlargement in the first weeks after creation but remaining stable thereafter [24–26,28,30]. Nishikawa et al. [14] and Gao et al. [24] demonstrated growth by means of maturation in rat venous pouch sidewall and bifurcation aneurysms. Fujiwara et al. [26] found a similar increase in size within the first four weeks with a further stable course of up to 4 months in an elastase arterial bifurcation stump model in rabbits. Naggara et al. [30] also found a maturation/growth within the first month and then stable course up to 10 months after creation of venous pouch terminal aneurysms in dogs. This may be explained by the absence of true perivascular inflammation and normal cellularity of the aneurysm walls. This healthy venous vascular tissue that the aneurysms were made of may have been able to organize to allow cell migration, and to synthesize a new extracellular matrix, eventually resulting in aneurysm healing. In contrast, the largest increase in size and true growth (ten-fold increase in size compared to baseline) was found in a rat abdominal aortic arterial pouch sidewall aneurysm model [8]. This remarkable growth was probably only possible due to aneurysm wall decellularization and the fact that the abdominal cavity is less restrictive than the subcutaneous soft tissue of the neck region.

More than half (55%) of the identified models demonstrated rupture of the experimental aneurysm during follow-up. In almost half of the reported models that demonstrate rupture, the aneurysm wall had been modified at the time of creation (Table 1). However, in all these models that featured rupture, the aneurysm wall was either weakened during creation (chemically or mechanically) or demonstrated marked wall degeneration (inflammation and intraluminal thrombosis) at autopsy. Stehbens [15] reported in 1979 that 30% (8/27) of venous sidewall aneurysms created at the common carotid artery in sheep ruptured within three weeks after creation. All these ruptured aneurysms contained macroscopic thrombus. Raymond et al. [3] demonstrated that 100% (7/7) of giant and 50% (2/4) of small-neck swine common carotid artery sidewall venous pouch aneurysms ruptured within 1–2 weeks after creation. They found that many areas of the aneurysm wall showed a lack of smooth muscle cells and elastic fibres but had inflammatory cells infiltrating the wall, along with hemorrhagic transformation of the media, adventitia, and perianeurysmal tissue. Yang et al. [29] presented a terminal rabbit aneurysm model with an arterial pouch modified with both elastase and collagenase. In this model, aneurysms grew within the first 1–2 weeks in 100% of cases (10/10) and 33% (3/9) of them ruptured within 4 weeks after creation. Histopathology revealed that the aneurysm wall was composed only of a thin layer of acellular fibrous tissue. Decellularization of the aneurysm wall in a sidewall rat aneurysm model resulted in aneurysm growth in 33% (4/12) and rupture in 25% (3/12) [8]. Decellularized aneurysms in this model demonstrated inflammation and damage to the aneurysm wall and marked neutrophil accumulation in the luminal thrombus.

In summary, loss of mural cells and chronic aneurysm wall inflammation is a crucial factor for both saccular aneurysm growth and rupture. It has been demonstrated that aneurysms that lost mural cells also lost their ability to organize luminal thrombus and to form a neointima [8,33]. Instead, ongoing inflammation results in destructive wall remodeling, further mural cell loss and thinning of the vascular wall which in turn favors further aneurysm growth and rupture. Thus, in order to establish a model which can reflect true aneurysm growth and rupture instead of just a short-term maturation, artificial rarefication of mural cells is necessary.

In addition to intracranial animal models for the study of aneurysm formation and rupture, it will be essential to further develop larger extracranial animal models that will allow to study embolization devices and healing processes in growing and rupture-prone aneurysms. Although most valuable, aneurysm models featuring growth and rupture are ethically questionable due to potential sudden death. Close monitoring (e.g., ultrasound imaging) to regularly check for the hemodynamic situation is recommended in all experimental aneurysm models featuring growth and rupture [3,8,34].

5. Conclusions

Extracranial saccular aneurysm models with growth and rupture are rare. Most of these models presented the increases in aneurysm size by means of maturation rather than ongoing degradation of the aneurysm wall and true growth that ultimately results in aneurysm rupture. Histological findings suggest that degradation of the wall (either by direct manipulation at the time of creation or indirect weakening mediated through intraluminal thrombosis and inflammation) is essential for rupture of an artificially created saccular aneurysm model. Since it has been shown that the aneurysm wall is important for healing after endovascular therapy, it is likely that models featuring growth and rupture will gain interest in the preclinical testing of novel endovascular therapies.

Funding: This study was supported by a research grant from the Kantonsspital Aarau, Aarau, Switzerland (FR 1400.000.054) and a grant from the Swiss National Science Foundation (SNSF 310030_182450/1).

Acknowledgments: We thank Erica Holt for editing.

Conflicts of Interest: The authors report no conflict of interests.

References

1. Alg, V.S.; Sofat, R.; Houlden, H.; Werring, D.J. Genetic risk factors for intracranial aneurysms: A meta-analysis in more than 116,000 individuals. *Neurology* **2013**, *80*, 2154–2165. [CrossRef] [PubMed]
2. Brinjikji, W.; Murad, M.H.; Lanzino, G.; Cloft, H.J.; Kallmes, D.F. Endovascular treatment of intracranial aneurysms with flow diverters: A meta-analysis. *Stroke J. Cereb. Circu.* **2013**, *44*, 442–447. [CrossRef] [PubMed]
3. Raymond, J.; Darsaut, T.E.; Kotowski, M.; Makoyeva, A.; Gevry, G.; Berthelet, F.; Salazkin, I. Thrombosis heralding aneurysmal rupture: An exploration of potential mechanisms in a novel giant swine aneurysm model. *Am. J. Neuroradiol.* **2013**, *34*, 346–353. [CrossRef] [PubMed]
4. Frösen, J.; Marjamaa, J.; Myllärniemi, M.; Abo-Ramadan, U.; Tulamo, R.; Niemelä, M.; Hernesniemi, J.; Jääskeläinen, J. Contribution of Mural and Bone Marrow-derived Neointimal Cells to Thrombus Organization and Wall Remodeling in a Microsurgical Murine Saccular Aneurysm Model. *Neurosurgery* **2006**, *58*, 936–944.
5. Frösen, J.; Tulamo, R.; Paetau, A.; Laaksamo, E.; Korja, M.; Laakso, A.; Niemelä, M.; Hernesniemi, J. Saccular intracranial aneurysm: Pathology and mechanisms. *Acta Neuropathol.* **2012**, *123*, 773–786.
6. Thompson, J.W.; Elwardany, O.; McCarthy, D.J.; Sheinberg, D.L.; Alvarez, C.M.; Nada, A.; Snelling, B.M.; Chen, S.H.; Sur, S.; Starke, R.M. In vivo cerebral aneurysm models. *Neurosurg. Focus* **2019**, *47*, E20. [CrossRef] [PubMed]
7. Marbacher, S.; Niemela, M.; Hernesniemi, J.; Frosen, J. Recurrence of endovascularly and microsurgically treated intracranial aneurysms-review of the putative role of aneurysm wall biology. *Neurosurg. Rev.* **2019**, *42*, 49–58. [CrossRef]

8. Marbacher, S.; Marjamaa, J.; Bradacova, K.; von Gunten, M.; Honkanen, P.; Abo-Ramadan, U.; Frösen, J. Loss of mural cells leads to wall degeneration, aneurysm growth, and eventual rupture in a rat aneurysm model. *Stroke J. Cereb. Circu.* **2014**, *45*, 248–254. [CrossRef]
9. Vanzin, J.; Mounayer, C.; Abud, D.G.; Annes, R.D.; Moret, J. Angiographic Results in Intracranial Aneurysms Treated with Inert Platinum Coils. *Interv. Neuroradiol.* **2012**, *18*, 391–400. [CrossRef]
10. Raymond, J.; Guilbert, F.; Weill, A.; Georganos, S.A.; Juravsky, L.; Lambert, A.; Lamoureux, J.; Chagnon, M.; Roy, D. Long-Term Angiographic Recurrences After Selective Endovascular Treatment of Aneurysms With Detachable Coils. *Stroke* **2003**, *34*, 1398–1403. [CrossRef]
11. Bouzeghrane, F.; Naggara, O.; Kallmes, D.F.; Berenstein, A.; Raymond, J.; International Consortium of Neuroendovascular Centres. In vivo experimental intracranial aneurysm models: A systematic review. *AJNR* **2010**, *31*, 418–423. [CrossRef] [PubMed]
12. Wang, S.; Dai, D.; Parameswaran, P.K.; Kadirvel, R.; Ding, Y.H.; Robertson, A.M.; Kallmes, D.F. Rabbit aneurysm models mimic histologic wall types identified in human intracranial aneurysms. *J. Neurointervent. Surg.* **2018**, *10*, 411–415. [CrossRef] [PubMed]
13. Troupp, H.; Rinne, T. Methyl-2-Cyanoacrylate (Eastman 910) in Experimental Vascular Surgery with a Note on Experimental Arterial Aneurysms. *J. Neurosurg.* **1964**, *21*, 1067–1069. [CrossRef] [PubMed]
14. Nishikawa, M.; Yonekawa, Y.; Matsuda, I. Experimental aneurysms. *Surg. Neurol.* **1976**, 5.
15. Stehbens, W.E. Chronic changes in the walls of experimentally produced aneurysms in sheep. *Surg. Gynecol. Obstet.* **1979**, *149*, 43–48.
16. Sadasivan, B.; Ma, S.; Dujovny, M.; Ho, K.L.; Ausman, J.I. Use of experimental aneurysms to evaluate wrapping materials. *Surg. Neurol.* **1990**, *34*, 3–7. [CrossRef]
17. Byrne, J.V.; Hubbard, N.; Morris, J.H. Endovascular coil occlusion of experimental aneurysms: Partial treatment does not prevent subsequent rupture. *Neurol. Res.* **1994**, *16*, 425–427. [CrossRef]
18. Raymond, J.; Venne, D.; Allas, S.; Roy, D.; Oliva, V.L.; Denbow, N.; Salazkin, I.; Leclerc, G. Healing mechanisms in experimental aneurysms. I. Vascular smooth muscle cells and neointima formation. *J. Neuroradiol.* **1999**, *26*, 7–20.
19. Yang, X.; Wu, Z.; Li, Y.; Tang, J.; Sun, Y.; Liu, Z.; Yin, K. Re-evaluation of cellulose acetate polymer: Angiographic findings and histological studies. *Surg. Neurol.* **2001**, *55*, 116–122. [CrossRef]
20. Becker, T.A.; Preul, M.C.; Bichard, W.D.; Kipke, D.R.; McDougall, C.G. PRELIMINARY INVESTIGATION OF CALCIUM ALGINATE GEL AS A BIOCOMPATIBLE MATERIAL FOR ENDOVASCULAR ANEURYSM EMBOLIZATION IN VIVO. *Neurosurgery* **2007**, *60*, 1119–1128. [CrossRef]
21. Ding, Y.H.; Tieu, T.; Kallmes, D.F. Creation of sidewall aneurysm in rabbits: Aneurysm patency and growth follow-up. *J. NeuroInterventional Surg.* **2012**, *6*, 29–31. [CrossRef] [PubMed]
22. Murayama, Y.; Tateshima, S.; Gonzalez, N.R.; Vinuela, F. Matrix and bioabsorbable polymeric coils accelerate healing of intracranial aneurysms: Long-term experimental study. *Stroke J. Cereb. Circul.* **2003**, *34*, 2031–2037. [CrossRef] [PubMed]
23. Young, P.H.; Fischer, V.W.; Guity, A.; Young, P.A. Mural repair following obliteration of aneurysms: Production of experimental aneurysms. *Microsurgure* **1987**, *8*, 128–137. [CrossRef] [PubMed]
24. Yong-Zhong, G.; August, H.; Van Alphen, M.; Kamphorst, W. Observations on experimental saccular aneurysms in the rat after 2 and 3 months. *Neurol. Res.* **1990**, *12*, 260–263. [CrossRef] [PubMed]
25. Kirse, D.J.; Flock, S.; Teo, C.; Rahman, S.; Mrak, R. Construction of a vein-pouch aneurysm at a surgically created carotid bifurcation in the rat. *Microsurgery* **1996**, *17*, 681–689. [CrossRef]
26. Fujiwara, N.H.; Cloft, H.J.; Marx, W.F.; Short, J.G.; E Jensen, M.; Kallmes, D.F. Serial angiography in an elastase-induced aneurysm model in rabbits: Evidence for progressive aneurysm enlargement after creation. *Am. J. Neuroradiol.* **2001**, 22.
27. Tsumoto, T.; Song, J.; Niimi, Y.; Berenstein, A. Interval Change in Size of Venous Pouch Canine Bifurcation Aneurysms over a 10-Month Period. *Am. J. Neuroradiol.* **2008**, *29*, 1067–1070. [CrossRef]
28. Graves, V.B.; Ahuja, A.; Strother, C.M.; Rappe, A.H. Canine model of terminal arterial aneurysm. *Am. J. Neuroradiol.* **1993**, 14.
29. Yang, X.-J.; Li, L.; Wu, Z.-x. A novel arterial pouch model of saccular aneurysm by concomitant elastase and collagenase digestion. *J. Zhejiang Univ. Sci.* **2007**, *8*, 697–703. [CrossRef]

30. Naggara, O.; Darsaut, T.E.; Salazkin, I.; Soulez, G.; Guilbert, F.; Roy, D.; Raymond, J. A new canine carotid artery bifurcation aneurysm model for the evaluation of neurovascular devices. *AJNR* **2010**, *31*, 967–971. [CrossRef]
31. McCune, W.S.; Samadi, A.; Blades, B. EXPERIMENTAL ANEURYSMS. *Ann. Surg.* **1953**, *138*, 216–218. [CrossRef] [PubMed]
32. White, J.C.; Sayre, G.P.; Whisnant, J.P. Experimental Destruction of the Media for the Production of Intracranial Arterial Aneurysms. *J. Neurosurg.* **1961**, *18*, 741–745. [CrossRef] [PubMed]
33. Marbacher, S.; Frosen, J.; Marjamaa, J.; Anisimov, A.; Honkanen, P.; Von Gunten, M.; Abo-Ramadan, U.; Hernesniemi, J.; Niemelä, M. Intraluminal Cell Transplantation Prevents Growth and Rupture in a Model of Rupture-Prone Saccular Aneurysms. *Stroke* **2014**, *45*, 3684–3690. [CrossRef] [PubMed]
34. Farnoush, A.; Avolio, A.; Qian, Y. A growth model of saccular aneurysms based on hemodynamic and morphologic discriminant parameters for risk of rupture. *J. Clin. Neurosci.* **2014**, *21*, 1514–1519. [CrossRef] [PubMed]

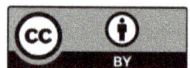

© 2020 by the authors. Licensee MDPI, Basel, Switzerland. This article is an open access article distributed under the terms and conditions of the Creative Commons Attribution (CC BY) license (http://creativecommons.org/licenses/by/4.0/).

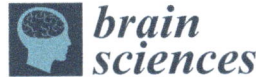

Case Report

Injury of Corticospinal Tract in a Patient with Subarachnoid Hemorrhage as Determined by Diffusion Tensor Tractography: A Case Report

Chan-Hyuk Park, Hyeong Ryu, Chang-Hwan Kim, Kyung-Lim Joa, Myeong-Ok Kim and Han-Young Jung *

Department of Physical & Rehabilitation Medicine, Inha University School of medicine, Inha University Hospital, Incheon 22332, Korea; chanhyuk@gmail.com (C.-H.P.); allen121212@naver.com (H.R.); jacob.kim@inha.ac.kr (C.-H.K.); drjoakl@gmail.com (K.-L.J.); rmkmo@inha.ac.kr (M.-O.K.)
* Correspondence: rmjung@inha.ac.kr; Tel.: +82-32-890-2480

Received: 15 February 2020; Accepted: 18 March 2020; Published: 19 March 2020

Abstract: We report diffusion tensor tractography (DTT) of the corticospinal tract (CST) in a patient with paresis of all four limbs following subarachnoid hemorrhage (SAH) with intraventricular hemorrhage (IVH) after the rupture of an anterior communicating artery (ACoA) aneurysm rupture. The 73-year-old female was admitted to our emergency room in a semi-comatose mental state. After coil embolization—an acute SAH treatment—she was transferred to our rehabilitation department with motor weakness development, two weeks after SAH. Upon admission, she was alert but she complained of motor weakness (upper limbs: MRC 3/5, and lower limbs: MRC 1/5). Four weeks after onset, DTT showed that the bilateral CSTs failed to reach the cerebral cortex. The left CST demonstrated a wide spread of fibers within the corona radiata as well as significantly lower tract volume (TV) and higher fractional anisotropy (FA) as well as mean diffusivity (MD) compared to the controls. On the other hand, the right CST shifted to the posterior region at the corona radiata, and MD values of the right CST were significantly higher when compared to the controls. Changes in both CSTs were attributed to vasogenic edema and compression caused by untreated hydrocephalus. We demonstrate in this case, two different pathophysiological entities, contributing to this patient's motor weakness after SAH.

Keywords: subarachnoid hemorrhage; ventriculomegaly; diffusion tensor imaging; corticospinal tract

1. Introduction

Anterior communicating artery (ACoA) aneurysms are the most common intracranial aneurysms and account for approximately 30% to 37% of subarachnoid hemorrhage (SAH) [1]. After aneurysm rupture, the resulting subarachnoid hemorrhage can result in complications such as cognition impairment [2]. However, motor weakness is also one of the neurological complications of SAH [3].

Many studies have used diffusion tensor tractography (DTT) to visualize neural tracts in the human brain, and as a result, DTT provides a useful means of evaluating neural tract injuries in human brain [4–6]. However, no DTT study has been performed examining the mechanisms responsible for motor weakness in the limbs of patients during the subacute phase following SAH with intraventricular hemorrhage (IVH). We hypothesize that, based on our DTT finding, that the injury of the corticospinal tract (CST) is due to SAH with intraventricular hemorrhage (IVH).

2. Case Presentation

A 73-year old female patient without a relevant prior medical history was admitted to our emergency room in a semi-comatose mental status (Glasgow Coma Scale: 3). Computed tomography

(CT) revealed a modified Fisher grade 4 SAH due to the rupture of a ACoA aneurysm, with consecutive hydrocephalus due to IVH (Figure 1A) [7]. After coil embolization, the patient was neurosurgically treated by hematoma evacuation and placement of an external ventricular drainage (EVD) (Figure 1B). Nimodipine was administered according to standing guidelines [8]. Two weeks after the initial ictus and upon improvement of her mental status, the patient was later transferred to our rehabilitation department. Upon admission, her mental status was altered, however, with reduced motor function of the upper and lower extremities (medical research council (MRC) grading of 3 in upper extremities and 1 in lower extremities). Bladder and bowel functions were preserved. We performed brain magnetic resonance imaging (MRI) at approximately week 4 after onset because of recovery of the CST within two weeks due to the resolution of peri-lesional edema or inflammation after stroke [9]. The result showed bilateral ventriculomegaly (Evan's index: 0.35) with ventricular capping, encephalomalacia in both frontal lobes, but no demarcated cerebral infarctions (Figure 2A).

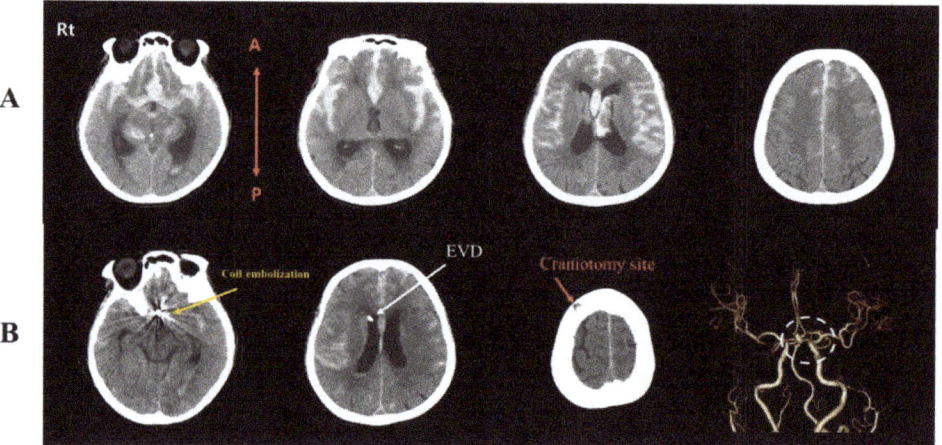

Figure 1. (**A**) Initial computed tomography (CT) images showing subarachnoid hemorrhage (SAH) with intraventricular hemorrhage (IVH) and consecutive ventriculomegaly, resulting from a ruptured anterior communicating artery aneurysm (ACoA). (**B**) CT image after coil embolization and external ventricular drainage (EVD) placement. Coil embolization (yellow arrow), EVD (white arrow), craniotomy site at the right frontal lobe (red arrow), and ACoA (white dashed circle). Note: EVD; external ventricular drainage, R, right; L, left; A, anterior; P, posterior.

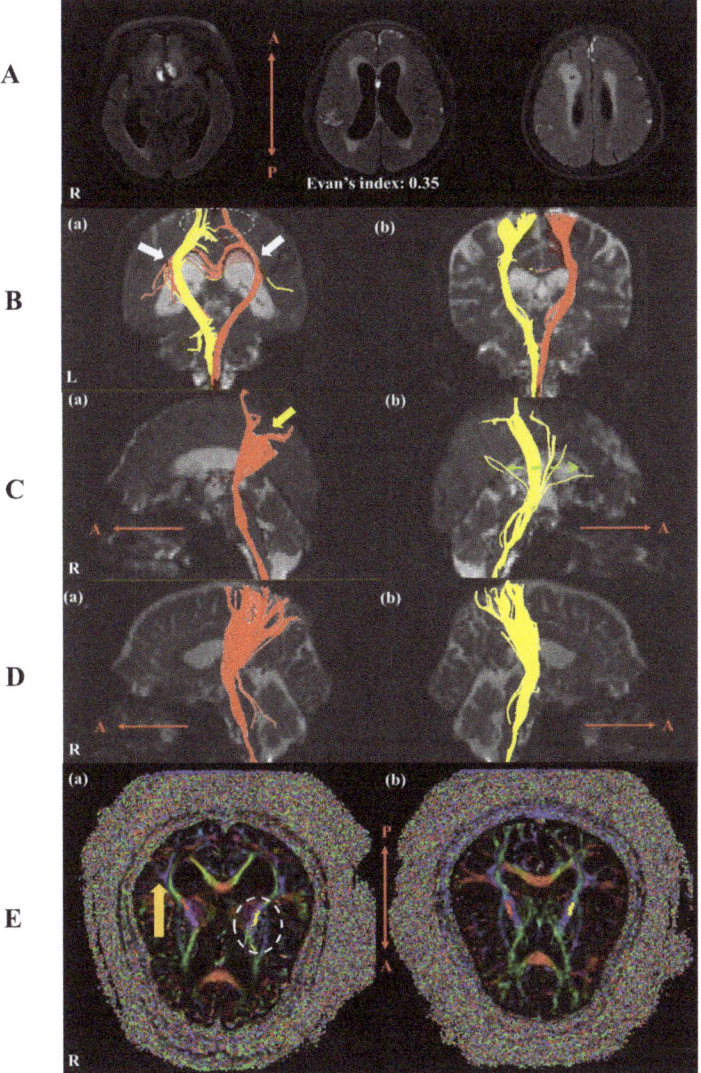

Figure 2. (**A**) Brain magnetic resonance images obtained at week 4 after onset showing clearance of subarachnoid blood with persisting bilateral ventriculomegaly (Evan's index: 0.35) with interstitial edema and encephalomalacia in both frontal lobes (severe enlargement of the left ventricle). (**B**) (a) Changes in both CSTs were observed around both lateral ventricles due to bilateral ventriculomegaly versus the control subjects (70 years old female, white arrow) and a discontinuity of both tracts to the bilateral cortex was apparent (white dash circle) (b) control. (**C**) (a) The right CST did not extend to the right cortex (yellow arrow) and (b) the left CST spread out (green dash arrow). (**D**) CSTs of a control subject. (**E**) (a) The right CST (red) was posteriorly shifted at the corona radiata (orange arrow) and the left CST (yellow) was spread out compared with control subjects (white dashed circle). (b) Left and right CSTs of a control subject. Note: R, right; L, left; A, anterior; P, posterior.

3. Diffusion Tensor Imaging

DTT images were obtained using a 3.0 T GE Signa Architect MRI System (General Electric, Milwaukee, WI, USA). The MRI preset conditions were as follows: field of view = 240×240 mm, acquisition matrix of 128×128, b = 1000 mm$^2 \cdot$s^{-1}, TR (repetition time) = 15,000 ms, TE (echo time) = 80.4 ms, slice thickness = 2 mm, 30 directions, and 72 contiguous slices. DTT images were analyzed using DTI studio software (www.mristudio.org, Johns Hopkins Medical Institute, Baltimore, USA). The CST was reconstructed using two regions of interest (ROIs). The seed ROIs were placed on the lower anterior pons and the target ROI was placed on the corona radiata. Termination criteria for fiber tracking were a fractional anisotropy (FA) of <0.2 and a turning angle of >60°. Mean diffusivities (MDs), tract volumes (TVs), and FAs of the CST tracks were measured. Results were compared with seven age-matched healthy control subjects (two males with a mean age of 70.14 years, age range 67–78 years) in this study. In prior analysis, we defined pathological changes as a deviation from reference values with at least two standard deviations [10]. At four weeks after onset, DTT revealed curved changes of both CSTs around both lateral ventricles due to bilateral ventriculomegaly compared with control subjects (Figure 2B). Furthermore, the right CST was shifted to the posterior region at the corona radiata without reaching the cerebral cortex, which was called the discontinuation (Figure 2B,C). The left CST appeared more spread out compared to the controls when looking at subcortical white matter and showed only a few fibers reaching the cerebral cortex (Figure 2B,C,E). FA and TV values of the left CST and MD values of both CSTs exhibited differences of two (SD) compared to our reference values (Table 1).

Table 1. Diffusion tensor tractography (DTT) parameter values of the corticospinal tracts of the patient and control subjects.

		FA	TV	MD ($\times 10^{-3}$ mm^2/s)
Patient	Right	0.632	3106.000	0.879 **
	Left	0.666 **	2148.000 **	0.763 **
Controls ($n = 7$)	Subject 1 (F/78)	0.617	3211.500	0.714
	Subject 2 (F/70)	0.598	2703.500	0.712
	Subject 3 (M/67)	0.623	2704.500	0.691
	Subject 4 (F/68)	0.612	2998.500	0.717
	Subject 5 (M/70)	0.633	3150.000	0.694
	Subject 6 (F/68)	0.624	3203.500	0.724
	Subject 7 (F/70)	0.607	3047.000	0.715
	Mean (SD)	0.616 (0.017)	3002.643 (218.341)	0.709 (0.012)

SD, standard deviation; F, female; M, male; CST, corticospinal tract; FA, fractional anisotropy; TV, tract volume; MD, mean diffusivity. ** Parameters were two SDs above or below mean normal control subject values.

4. Discussion

The corticospinal tract (CST) constitutes the main white matter motor pathway [11]. In this patient with generalized motor weakness after SAH, the CST was investigated using DTT MRI imaging. Bilateral CST reconstruction using DTT revealed side-dependent differences between our subject in comparison to a matched cohort of control patients. More specifically, changes in CST structures were observed around the corona radiata and lateral ventricle; the right CST had moved posteriorly and the left CST was spread out at the level of the corona radiata, compared to the healthy controls. Apart from displacement, the CSTs revealed signs of discontinuation at the cerebral cortex. Furthermore, in the left CST, the FA and MD values were elevated and TV values reduced, and in the right CST, the MD values were alerted due to a greater or lower difference than two standard deviations compared with the control subjects.

FA values represent degrees of directionality at a microscopic level [10,12,13], and thus provide a means of assessing microstructural integrity of axons, myelin, and microtubules [4,14]. On the other hand, MD values provide quantitative measures of water diffusion, and are indicative of pathological changes taking place in white matter [15]. Increases in the values of MD represent vasogenic edema or axonal damage whereas a decrease in MD values indicates neural injury [16]. TV values represent numbers of voxels within neural tracts [16]. Therefore, FA and TV reductions in combination with MD increases indicate the presence of neural injury [6,16].

In a previous study, it was reported that patients with normal pressure hydrocephalus (NPH) had initial high FA values, explained by mechanical compression and decreased FA and increased MD values as a result of secondary degenerative changes [3,17,18]. In this case, our patient exhibited bilateral displacement and discontinuation of CSTs before reaching the cerebral cortex. In addition, our MR imaging revealed high FA and MD values in combination with low TV value in the left CST. However, the FA value of the right CST was not increased significantly. Based on these findings, we hypothesized that the mechanism of motor weakness in our case was different between sides. At week 4 after onset, posterior displacement of the right CST, as the result of hydrocephalus caused ventriculomegaly, resulted in a discontinuation of the tract to the cerebral cortex. Significantly high MD values were found with the number of voxels contained within neural tracts and FA values remaining unchanged. We believed that the changes to the right CST are mainly caused by vasogenic edema without neural injury, leading to the discontinuation of the tract resulting loss of left motor function. In contrast to our results during the subacute phage, a previous study reported the formation of vasogenic edema following SAH in the acute phase [19]. Further MRI assessment of the timely development of vasogenic edema after SAH is necessary. However, in the left CST, spreading within the corona radiata was observed due to ventriculomegaly caused mechanical compression. This, based on the observed increased FA values, decreased TV, and increased MD indicative of degenerative change or neural tract injury. These observations led to the paralysis of right limbs. However, we were able to exclude age-associated microstructural changes because while age-associated microstructural changes using DTT showed increased FA and MD values, our patient reveal no reduced FA value [20]. Additionally, as a previous study, the analysis of CST for upper and lower limbs using DTT is difficult due to the discontinuation of CSTs at the cerebral cortex [21]. However, we believe that a few fibers to the cerebral cortex could play a role in upper motor function and tracts associated with lower motor function were injured due to a compression of lateral ventricle and their discontinuation. However, the defined causes of mechanical compression on the left side there and vasogenic edema in the right side were not defined as effects at four weeks after SAH, so further study is required.

Therefore, at four weeks after onset (subacute phase), injury of the left tracts resulted from degenerative change of the tracts (increased MD value and decreased TV value) and mechanical compression (increased FA value). Damage to the right CST caused vasogenic edema by ventriculomegaly. We believe that because of the larger left ventricle, mechanical compression had greater influence on the left CST in terms of increasing FA. In other words, we indicate that mechanical compression and degenerative changes by ventriculomegaly can coexist and induce tract injury. In addition, we believe that the right CST injury resulted from vasogenic edema based on differences in morphology of the tract caused by the difference in ventricle size.

The most feared complication following SAH is delayed cerebral ischemia. To prevent delayed cerebral ischemia, our patient administrated aspirin and cilostazol [8]. Another complication is hydrocephalus [7]. The patient received an EVD during the acute phase and was constantly being monitored for persisting hydrocephalus. Previous studies have also presented mechanisms of motor weakness after SAH or NPH [3,17]. It has been suggested that one of the mechanisms of paraplegia or paraparesis after SAH is hydrocephalus [3]. However, to the best of our knowledge, this case report is the first to observe a side-dependent different mechanism resulting in motor weakness as a result of asymmetrical hydrocephalic ventriculomegaly (mechanical compression at the left hemisphere and vasogenic edema at the right hemisphere). However, this study has some limitations, as follows: (1) The external validity of these observations remains limited because they are based on a single case, larger scale long-term studies are necessary to confirm our hypothesis; (2) As our study was in the subacute phase, long-term follow up is necessary; (3) DTT interpretation is operator-dependent, leading to potential performance bias [11]; and (4) Finally, further clarification via electrophysiological examination of long fiber tracts would have been helpful, but was hindered due to the existing craniotomy defect [22].

5. Conclusions

Although DTT is subjected to operator-dependency [11], we can conclude a coexistence of side-dependent compressive and degenerative damage to the CST caused by either ventriculomegaly or direct compression, leading to bilateral motor weakness. Here, DTT was proven to be a useful tool in assessing the mechanism behind post-SAH persisting motor weakness.

Author Contributions: Conceptualization, C.-H.P. and H.-Y.J.; Methodology, C.-H.P. and K.-L.J.; Software, C.-H.P.; Formal analysis, C.-H.P. and H.-Y.J.; Investigation, H.R. and C.-H.P.; Data curation, H.R. and C.-H.P; Writing—original draft preparation, C.-H.P.; Writing—review and editing, C.-H.K., K.-L.J., and H.-Y.J.; Supervision, M.-O.K. and H.-Y.J.; Project administration, H.-Y.J. All authors have read and agreed to the published version of the manuscript.

Funding: This research received no external funding.

Conflicts of Interest: The authors declare no conflicts of interest.

References

1. Andaluz, N.; Zuccarello, M. Anterior Communicating Artery Aneurysm Surgery through the Orbitopterional Approach: Long-Term Follow-Up in a Series of 75 Consecutive Patients. *Skull Base.* **2008**, *18*, 265–274. [CrossRef]
2. Mavaddat, N.; Sahakian, B.; Hutchinson, P.J.; Kirkpatrick, P.J. Cognition following subarachnoid hemorrhage from anterior communicating artery aneurysm: Relation to timing of surgery. *J. Neurosurg.* **1999**, *91*, 402–407. [CrossRef]
3. Jang, S.H.; Lee, H. Do the pathogenic mechanisms of motor weakness following aneurysmal subarachnoid hemorrhage: A review. *Neurol. Asia* **2017**, *22*, 185–191.
4. Jang, S.H.; Seo, J.P. Differences of the medial lemniscus and spinothalamic tract according to the cortical termination areas: A diffusion tensor tractography study. *Somatosens. Mot. Res.* **2014**, *32*, 67–71. [CrossRef]
5. Son, S.M.; Kim, J.H. Activation of less affected corticospinal tract and poor motor outcome in hemiplegic pediatric patients: A diffusion tensor tractography imaging study. *Neural Regen. Res.* **2015**, *10*, 2054–2059. [CrossRef]
6. Jang, S.H.; Seo, Y.S. Diagnosis of Conversion Disorder Using Diffusion Tensor Tractography and Transcranial Magnetic Stimulation in a Patient with Mild Traumatic Brain Injury. *Diagnostics* **2019**, *9*, 155. [CrossRef]
7. Danière, F.; Gascou, G.; De Champfleur, N.M.; Machi, P.; Leboucq, N.; Riquelme, C.; Ruiz, C.; Bonafe, A.; Costalat, V. Complications and follow up of subarachnoid hemorrhages. *Diagn. Interv. Imaging* **2015**, *96*, 677–686. [CrossRef]
8. Oppong, M.D.; Gembruch, O.; Pierscianek, D.; Köhrmann, M.; Kleinschnitz, C.; Deuschl, C.; Mönninghoff, C.; Kaier, K.; Forsting, M.; Sure, U.; et al. Post-treatment Antiplatelet Therapy Reduces Risk for Delayed Cerebral Ischemia due to Aneurysmal Subarachnoid Hemorrhage. *Neurosurgery* **2018**, *85*, 827–833. [CrossRef]
9. Jang, S.H. The role of the corticospinal tract in motor recovery in patients with a stroke: A review. *NeuroRehabilitation* **2009**, *24*, 285–290. [CrossRef]
10. Yeo, S.S.; Jang, S.H.; Lee, J. Central post-stroke pain due to injury of the spinothalamic tract in patients with cerebral infarction: A diffusion tensor tractography imaging study. *Neural Regen. Res.* **2017**, *12*, 2021–2024. [CrossRef]
11. Jang, S.H.; Kim, S.H.; Jang, W.H. Recovery of corticospinal tract injured by traumatic axonal injury at the subcortical white matter: A case report. *Neural Regen. Res.* **2016**, *11*, 1527–1528. [CrossRef]
12. Neil, J.J. Diffusion imaging concepts for clinicians. *J. Magn. Reson. Imaging* **2007**, *27*, 1–7. [CrossRef]
13. O'Donnell, L.J.; Westin, C.-F. An Introduction to Diffusion Tensor Image Analysis. *Neurosurg. Clin. North Am.* **2011**, *22*, 185–196. [CrossRef]

14. Santillo, A.F.; Mårtensson, J.; Lindberg, O.; Nilsson, M.; Manzouri, A.; Waldö, M.L.; Van Westen, D.; Wahlund, L.-O.; Latt, J.; Nilsson, C. Diffusion Tensor Tractography versus Volumetric Imaging in the Diagnosis of Behavioral Variant Frontotemporal Dementia. *Plos ONE* **2013**, *8*, e66932. [CrossRef]
15. Koyama, T.; Marumoto, K.; Domen, K.; Ohmura, T.; Miyake, H. Diffusion tensor imaging of idiopathic normal pressure hydrocephalus: A voxel-based fractional anisotropy study. *Neurol. Medico-Chirurgica* **2012**, *52*, 68–74. [CrossRef]
16. Jang, S.H.; Seo, J.P.; Lee, S.J. Diffusion Tensor Tractography Studies of Central Post-stroke Pain Due to the Spinothalamic Tract Injury: A Mini-Review. *Front. Neurol.* **2019**, *10*, 787. [CrossRef]
17. Hoza, D.; Vlasak, A.; Hořínek, D.; Sameš, M.; Alfieri, A. DTI-MRI biomarkers in the search for normal pressure hydrocephalus aetiology: A review. *Neurosurg. Rev.* **2014**, *38*, 239–244. [CrossRef]
18. Nakanishi, A.; Fukunaga, I.; Hori, M.; Masutani, Y.; Takaaki, H.; Miyajima, M.; Aoki, S. Microstructural changes of the corticospinal tract in idiopathic normal pressure hydrocephalus: A comparison of diffusion tensor and diffusional kurtosis imaging. *Neuroradiol.* **2013**, *55*, 971–976. [CrossRef]
19. Weimer, J.; Jones, S.; Frontera, J. Acute Cytotoxic and Vasogenic Edema after Subarachnoid Hemorrhage: A Quantitative MRI Study. *Am. J. Neuroradiol.* **2017**, *38*, 928–934. [CrossRef]
20. Pareek, V.; Rallabandi, V.S.; Prasun, R. A Correlational Study between Microstructural White Matter Properties and Macrostructural Gray Matter Volume across Normal Ageing: Conjoint DTI and VBM Analysis. *Magn. Reson. Insights* **2018**, *11*, 1178623. [CrossRef]
21. Kwon, H.G.; Hong, J.-H.; Jang, S.H. Anatomic Location and Somatotopic Arrangement of the Corticospinal Tract at the Cerebral Peduncle in the Human Brain. *Am. J. Neuroradiol.* **2011**, *32*, 2116–2119. [CrossRef] [PubMed]
22. Legatt, A.D.; Emerson, R.G.; Epstein, C.M.; Macdonald, D.B.; Deletis, V.; Bravo, R.J.; Lopez, J.R. ACNS Guideline. *J. Clin. Neurophysiol.* **2016**, *33*, 42–50. [CrossRef] [PubMed]

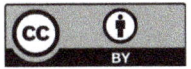

© 2020 by the authors. Licensee MDPI, Basel, Switzerland. This article is an open access article distributed under the terms and conditions of the Creative Commons Attribution (CC BY) license (http://creativecommons.org/licenses/by/4.0/).

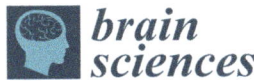 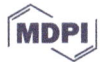

Case Report

Syncope as Initial Presentation in an Undifferentiated Type Acute Myeloid Leukemia Patient with Acute Intracranial Hemorrhage

Meng-Yu Wu [1,2], Ching-Hsiang Lin [1,2], Yueh-Tseng Hou [1,2], Po-Chen Lin [1,2], Giou-Teng Yiang [1,2], Yueh-Cheng Tien [1,2,*] and Hsiao-Ching Yeh [3,*]

1. Department of Emergency Medicine, Taipei Tzu Chi Hospital, Buddhist Tzu Chi Medical Foundation, New Taipei 231, Taiwan
2. Department of Emergency Medicine, School of Medicine, Tzu Chi University, Hualien 970, Taiwan
3. Psychiatry Department, Chang Bing Show-Chwan Memorial Hospital, Changhua 505, Taiwan
* Correspondence: artist0310@gmail.com (Y.-C.T.); olive01478963@gmail.com (H.-C.Y.); Tel.: +886-2-6628-9779 (Y.-C.T.); Fax: +886-2-6628-9009 (Y.-C.T.)

Received: 24 July 2019; Accepted: 17 August 2019; Published: 20 August 2019

Abstract: Intracranial hemorrhage (ICH) is a catastrophic complication in patients with acute myeloid leukemia (AML). AML cells, especially in the acute promyelocytic leukemia subtype, may release microparticles (MPs), tissue factor (TF), and cancer procoagulant (CP) to promote coagulopathy. Hyperfibrinolysis is also triggered via release of annexin II, t-PA, u-PA, and u-PAR. Various inflammatory cytokines from cancer cells, such as IL-1β and TNF-α, activate endothelial cells and promote leukostasis. This condition may increase the ICH risk and lead to poor clinical outcomes. Here, we present a case under a unique situation with acute ICH detected prior to the diagnosis of AML. The patient initially presented with two episodes of syncope. Rapidly progressive ICH was noted in follow-up computed tomography (CT) scans. Therefore, we highlight that AML should be among the differential diagnoses of the etiologies of ICH. Early diagnosis and timely intervention are very important for AML patients.

Keywords: syncope; acute myeloid leukemia; intracranial hemorrhage; hyperleukocytosis; blast crisis

1. Introduction

Intracranial hemorrhage (ICH) is an uncommon complication in patients with acute myeloid leukemia (AML), and coincides with poor clinical outcome. The mortality rate of AML patients developing acute ICH is high and death can occur within days if not diagnosed and treated appropriately. In a study by Owattanapanich et al. [1], 4.29% (38/685 patients) AML patients presented with ICH and acute promyelocytic leukemia had a higher risk of ICH with odds ratio of 6.15, compared to other types in the AML subgroup analysis [1]. Few patients with acute myeloid leukemia in undifferentiated type presented syncope and ICH as an initial presentation. AML with undifferentiated type (AML-M1) patients were presented with ICH accounting for only 15.79% (6/38 patients). In addition, only 10% of patients present hyperleukocytosis, which are at higher risk of tumor lysis syndrome and leukostasis [2]. Several risk factors were investigated, including hypertension, vasculopathy, thrombocytopenia, lower coagulation factors, disseminated intravascular coagulation (DIC), and hyperleukocytosis. Hyperleukocytosis and DIC were two major factors associated with ICH. The incidence of hyperleukocytosis in acute AML patients was 5–20% and this condition may be significantly associated with DIC, leukostasis, and tumor lysis syndrome, promoting ICH events. However, clinical experiences concerning ICH in AML are limited in the literature. Therefore, early diagnosis and timely intervention are crucial for AML patients. Here, we describe a rare case of syncope at initial presentation in an AML-M0 patient with acute intracranial hemorrhage.

2. Case Presentation

This case report was approved by the Institutional Review Board of Taipei Tzu Chi Hospital, Buddhist Tzu Chi Medical Foundation (IRB number: 08-CR-060).

A 31-year-old male presented with a productive cough and rhinorrhea for 4 days. He had no past medical history or medicine history. The symptoms were associated with intermittent high fever up to 39–40 °C and myalgia. He took symptomatic treatment but in vain. The patient went to a local medical doctor for treatment. While waiting outside the consulting room, syncope occurred twice and he contused the frontal area. There was no tonic or clonic seizure. Other symptoms, including skin rash, arthritis, or tendency for abnormal bleeding, were not found. Pneumonia-induced sepsis was suspected, and he was transferred to our emergency department. Upon admission, his temperature was 38.4 °C, blood pressure was 110/62 mmHg, heart rate was 129 beats/min, body weight was 90.6 kg, and height was 173 cm. Upon physical examination, his Glasgow Coma Score (GCS) score was E4V5M6 and bilateral pupil size was 2 mm with light reflex. There was no horizontal or vertical nystagmus. The neck was supple with no limited range of motion. The bilateral breath sound was clear without wheezing or crackle, and tachycardia was noted. There was no Babinski sign, decreased muscle power, or unsteady gait. The chest X-ray revealed no significant pulmonary nodules or pneumonia patch. An influenza A + B rapid screening test was performed, which showed negative results. A brain CT revealed a 13 mm lesion with hyperdensity in the left temporal region, with suspected intracerebral hemorrhage (Figure 1). Laboratory evaluation of the patient revealed severe leukocytosis with blastemia (Table 1).

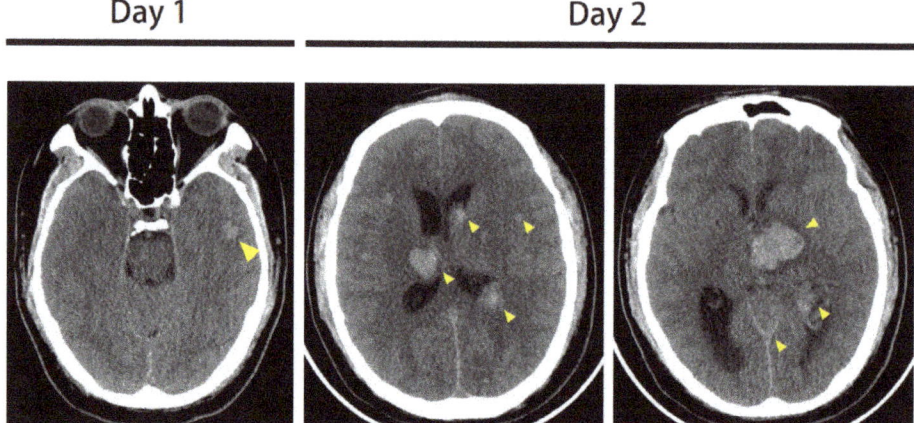

Figure 1. On the day 1 brain computed tomography (CT), a 13 mm lesion with hyperdensity was found in the left temporal region, with suspected intracerebral hemorrhage. On the day 2 brain CT, multifocal intracranial hemorrhages in bilateral cerebral hemispheres were noted, the largest being a 30 mm lesion in the left thalamus. The midline structures were shifted to the right side. Extensive swelling was present in the cerebellum and brain stem.

Table 1. The laboratory evaluation in this patient.

Variables	Normal Range	Patient Data			
		Day 1	Day 2	Day 3	Day 4
White cell count	3.5–11 × 10^9/L	56.1	54.6	51.3	59.0
Band form neutrophils	0–3%	0.0%	0.0%	0.0%	0.0%
Segment form neutrophils	45–70%	0.0%	0.0%	0.0%	0.0%
Lymphocytes	25–40%	16.0%	7.0%	4.0%	6.0%
Eosinophils	1–3%	0.0%	0.0%	0.0%	0.0%
Monocytes	2–8%	6.0%	0.0%	0.0%	0.0%
Basophils	0–1%	0.0%	0.0%	0.0%	0.0%
Myelocytes	0.0%	0.0%	1.0%	0.0%	1.0%
Nucleated red blood cells	0.0%	0.0%	0.0%	0.0%	3.0%
Blast	0.0%	84.0%	92.0%	96.0%	93.0%
Hemoglobin	7.45–9.93 mmoL/L	5.40	4.65	4.47	5.28
Platelet counts	150–400 × 10^9/L	64	54	146	130
Blood urine nitrogen	2.5–6.4 mmoL/L	7.5	7.9	7.1	—-
Creatinine	0.04–0.09 mmoL/L	0.168	0.1591	0.1591	—-
Sodium	136–145 mmoL/L	138	144	157	147
Potassium	3.5–5.1 mmoL/L	2.8	2.2	4.1	2.7
Glucose	3.9–5.6 mmoL/L	6.3	—-	—-	—-
Alanine aminotransferase	0.27–1.05 μkat/L	0.50	—-	0.55	—-
High-sensitive Troponin I	0–19 ng/L	82.1	—-	—-	—-
C-Reactive Protein	<31.4 nmoL/L	810.5	—-	—-	—-
Prothrombin time	8.0–12.0 s	12.7	12.1	12.7	—-
Partial thromboplastin time	23.9–35.5 s	26.8	26.5	25.0	—-
FDP-Ddimer	0–500 μg/L	708.18	552.51	—-	—-

Results from the bone marrow biopsy report showed 90% cellularity. Blasts accounted for more than 90% of all nucleated cells. Hypercellular and monotonous bone marrow was noted with undifferentiated myeloblasts with prominent, convoluted nuclei, and agranular cytoplasm. There were significantly decreased erythroid and megakaryocyte lineages. The immunohistochemical profile was as follows: CD34(+), CD117(+), MPO(+), CD33(+), CD68(−), hemoglobin A(−), Factor VIII(−), CD19(−), CD3(−), TdT(−), and PAX5(−). The peroxidase and alpha naphthyl acetate esterase (ANAE) test was positive and chloroacetate esterase (CAE) test was negative. Acute myeloid leukemia was diagnosed. Broad-spectrum antibiotic and adequate hydration were administered. An antineoplastic agent, hydroxyurea (15 mg/kg/day), and emergency leukocytapheresis were used to control disease progression. Unfortunately, the patient became drowsy with asymmetric pupil size and no light reflex. The follow-up brain CT showed multifocal intracranial hemorrhage in the bilateral cerebral hemispheres with midline shift involving the brain stem (Figure 1). Progressive hypotension was noted even using a vasopressor agent. Finally, the patient expired due to uncontrolled hemodynamic shock on the fourth day.

3. Discussion

In the AML population, intracranial-hemorrhage-induced syncope at initial presentation is an uncommon but fatal condition. The study by Balmages et al. [3] showed a similar AML case with hyperleukocytosis (WBC count of 51.7 × 10^9/L) was reported. In those populations, there was a significantly higher risk of death from rapidly developed fatal ICH. In the study by Chen et al. [4], a total of 841 AML patients were enrolled, and 6% (51/841 patients) were diagnosed with ICH. The location of ICH was common at supratentorium (44/51 cases), followed by basal ganglion (9/51 cases), cerebellum (5/51 cases), and brainstem (4/51 cases). The analysis of clinical outcome revealed that 67% of patients (34 patients) died of ICH within 30 days of diagnosis. Severe DIC and leukostasis are two main causes leading to ICH. In the untreated AML population, 5–20% of patients may present with hyperleukocytosis, defined by white blood cell counts > 100,000/mL [5,6]. The hyperleukocytosis may result from a rapid blast proliferation and hematopoietic cell adhesion dysfunction [7]. Hyperleukocytosis may induce DIC, tumor lysis syndrome, and leukostasis. The brain and lungs are the common organs involved, and are associated with a high mortality rate. Severe hyperleukocytosis may induce mechanical obstruction of small vessels, causing malperfusion, endothelial damage, subsequent hemorrhage, and cell death [8]. The mechanical obstruction may be induced by myeloblasts via release of various inflammatory cytokines and factors, such as IL-1β and TNF-α, to promote endothelial cell activation [9]. The activated endothelial cells increase the expression of adhesion receptors, such as intracellular adhesion molecule-1 (ICAM-1) and vascular cell adhesion molecule-1 (VCAM-1) (Figure 2). However, cytokine-driven endothelial cell activation, which is induced by AML, may lead to a loss of vascular integrity and impaired endothelial antithrombotic function [10,11]. The endothelial damage can then lead to impaired myeloblast migration and subsequent hemorrhage.

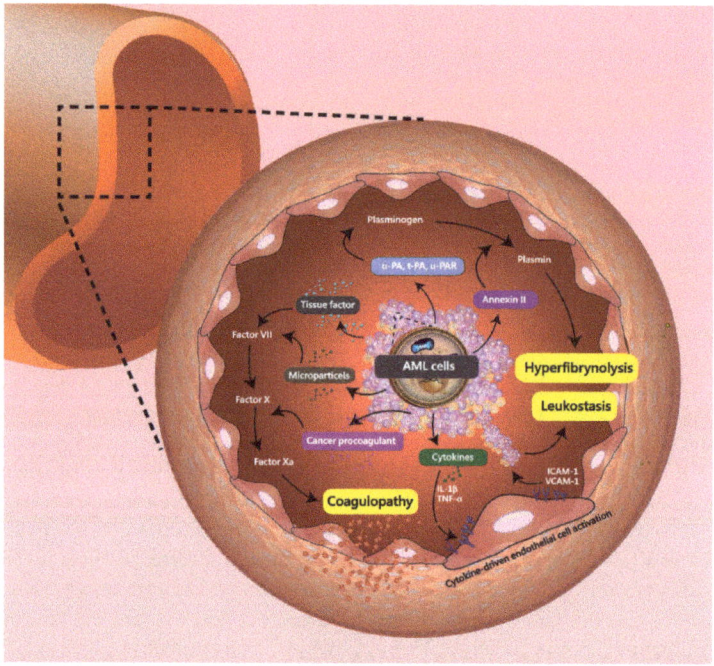

Figure 2. In an APL model, the acute myeloid leukemia (AML) cell produces microparticles (MPs), tissue factor (TF), and cancer procoagulant (CP), which act on the coagulation cascade to promote coagulopathy. The release of annexin II, t-PA, u-PA, and u-PAR from AML cells converts plasminogen into plasmin, causing hyperfibrinolysis. Various inflammatory cytokines from cancer cells, such as IL-1β and TNF-α, also activate endothelial cells and promote leukostasis.

In the study by Dixit et al. [12], DIC was found in 16.6% of AML patients (4/24 patients; M2: 1 case, M3: 2 cases, M5: 1 case). Acute promyelocytic leukemia is a subtype of AML, characterized by fatal bleeding events, and has also been well investigated [13]. Coagulopathy may be induced by AML cells via high expression of tissue factor, activating the coagulation cascade. In an APL model, the cells expressed high levels of three main procoagulants, including microparticles (MPs), tissue factor (TF), and cancer procoagulant (CP) [14]. TF is a cell surface receptor that catalyzes the conversion of factor X into factor Xa through factor VIIa. CP is a cysteine protease procoagulant involving the coagulation cascade by activating factor X to promote thrombin [15]. MPs decrease coagulation time in AML and promote coagulopathy via increased thrombin generation [16]. High levels of annexin II, t-PA, u-PA, and u-PAR were also found to activate plasminogen into plasmin in AML cells, which induced hyperfibrinolysis [17,18]. In addition, endothelial cells may be destroyed via release of various inflammatory cytokines, such as IL-1β and TNF-α, to promote DIC (Figure 2) [19].

Leukapheresis in AML patients with hyperleukocytosis rapidly removes excessive leukocytes by mechanical separation to control complications. One round of leukapheresis could reduce the WBC count by about 10–70% [20]. The efficacy of leukapheresis has been reported in previous clinical trials, but there are some trials that disagree. After leukapheresis, AML cells may rapidly mobilize from the bone marrow to peripheral blood. In addition, the benefit of leukapheresis was not significant in clinical trials and the long-term outcome was not changed. However, leukapheresis may be beneficial for preventing leukostasis and reducing the risk of ICH. A study by Novotny et al. [21] included 95 hyperleukocytic leukemia patients and evaluated the effectiveness of therapy using the four-stage clinical grading scale. The results showed that the AML M1/M2 population with hyperleukocytosis ($p = 0.011$), lower hemoglobin ($p = 0.004$), and blast crisis ($p = 0.004$) presented with highly probable leukostasis with a high score. A subgroup was given early leukapheresis treatment which showed a benefit (based on a grading score) in preventing leukostasis-related early death. In our case, hyperleukocytosis with thrombocytopenia and blast crisis was noted. Leukapheresis was performed but the treatment was not very effective. Persistent leukostasis and DIC promoted the progression of ICH with multiple focal hemorrhages in day 2 CT scans.

4. Conclusions

In this article, we present the rare and unusual case of a patient with AML-induced ICH initially presenting with syncope. In the AML population, DIC and leukostasis play a critical role in ICH. This detailed pathophysiology may improve physicians' development of therapeutic strategies for AML-induced ICH. Here, we highlight the clinical features and etiologies of AML-induced ICH. Early diagnosis and timely leukapheresis may prevent fatal progressive complications.

Author Contributions: M.-Y.W. and C.-H.L., wrote the paper; G.-T.Y., Y.-T.H., and P.-C.L., contributed to the organization of the figures; G.-T.Y. and Y.-T.H., provided conceptual input; Y.-C.T. and H.-C.Y., proofread and organized the manuscript. All authors reviewed the final version of the manuscript.

Funding: This study was supported by a grant from Taipei Tzu Chi Hospital (TCRD-TPE-108-5).

Acknowledgments: In this section you can acknowledge any support given which is not covered by the author contribution or funding sections. This may include administrative and technical support, or donations in kind (e.g., materials used for experiments).

Conflicts of Interest: The authors declare no conflict of interest.

References

1. Owattanapanich, W.; Auewarakul, C.U. Intracranial Hemorrhage in Patients with Hematologic Disorders: Prevalence and Predictive Factors. *J. Med. Assoc. Thai.* **2016**, *99*, 15–24. [PubMed]
2. Jabbour, E.J.; Estey, E.; Kantarjian, H.M. Adult Acute Myeloid Leukemia. *Mayo. Clin. Proc.* **2006**, *81*, 247–260. [CrossRef] [PubMed]
3. Balmages, A.; Dinglasan, J.; Osborn, M.B. Severe Intracranial Hemorrhage at Initial Presentation of Acute Myelogenous Leukemia. *Clin. Pract. Cases Emerg. Med.* **2018**, *2*, 203–206. [CrossRef] [PubMed]
4. Chen, C.Y.; Tai, C.H.; Tsay, W.; Chen, P.Y.; Tien, H.F. Prediction of Fatal Intracranial Hemorrhage in Patients with Acute Myeloid Leukemia. *Ann. Oncol.* **2009**, *20*, 1100–1104. [CrossRef] [PubMed]
5. Pastore, F.; Pastore, A.; Wittmann, G.; Hiddemann, W.; Spiekermann, K. The Role of Therapeutic Leukapheresis in Hyperleukocytotic Aml. *PLoS ONE* **2014**, *9*, e95062. [CrossRef] [PubMed]
6. Ventura, G.J.; Hester, J.P.; Smith, T.L.; Keating, M.J. Acute Myeloblastic Leukemia with Hyperleukocytosis: Risk Factors for Early Mortality in Induction. *Am. J. Hematol.* **1988**, *27*, 34–37. [CrossRef] [PubMed]
7. Reuss-Borst, M.A.; Klein, G.; Waller, H.D.; Muller, C.A. Differential Expression of Adhesion Molecules in Acute Leukemia. *Leukemia* **1995**, *9*, 869–874. [PubMed]
8. Rollig, C.; Ehninger, G. How I Treat Hyperleukocytosis in Acute Myeloid Leukemia. *Blood* **2015**, *125*, 3246–3252. [CrossRef]

9. Stucki, A.; Rivier, A.S.; Gikic, M.; Monai, N.; Schapira, M.; Spertini, O. Endothelial Cell Activation by Myeloblasts: Molecular Mechanisms of Leukostasis and Leukemic Cell Dissemination. *Blood* **2001**, *97*, 2121–2129. [CrossRef]
10. Hunt, B.J.; Jurd, K.M. Endothelial Cell Activation. A Central Pathophysiological Process. *BMJ* **1998**, *316*, 1328–1329. [CrossRef]
11. Mantovani, A.; Sozzani, S.; Vecchi, A.; Introna, M.; Allavena, P. Cytokine Activation of Endothelial Cells: New Molecules for an Old Paradigm. *Thromb. Haemost.* **1997**, *78*, 406–414. [CrossRef]
12. Dixit, A.; Chatterjee, T.; Mishra, P.; Kannan, M.; Choudhry, D.R.; Mahapatra, M.; Choudhry, V.P.; Saxena, R. Disseminated Intravascular Coagulation in Acute Leukemia at Presentation and During Induction Therapy. *Clin. Appl. Thromb. Hemost.* **2007**, *13*, 292–298. [CrossRef]
13. Kuchenbauer, F.; Buske, C. Revisiting Thrombocytopenia in Acute Promyelocytic Leukemia. *Leukemia* **2018**, *32*, 1477–1478. [CrossRef]
14. David, S.; Mathews, V. Mechanisms and Management of Coagulopathy in Acute Promyelocytic Leukemia. *Thromb. Res.* **2018**, *164*, S82–88. [CrossRef]
15. Wang, J.; Weiss, I.; Svoboda, K.; Kwaan, H.C. Thrombogenic Role of Cells Undergoing Apoptosis. *Br. J. Haematol.* **2001**, *115*, 382–391. [CrossRef]
16. Ma, G.; Liu, F.; Lv, L.; Gao, Y.; Su, Y. Increased Promyelocytic-Derived Microparticles: A Novel Potential Factor for Coagulopathy in Acute Promyelocytic Leukemia. *Ann. Hematol.* **2013**, *92*, 645–652. [CrossRef]
17. Tapiovaara, H.; Alitalo, R.; Stephens, R.; Myohanen, H.; Ruutu, T.; Vaheri, A. Abundant Urokinase Activity on the Surface of Mononuclear Cells from Blood and Bone Marrow of Acute Leukemia Patients. *Blood* **1993**, *82*, 914–919.
18. Nadir, Y.; Katz, T.; Sarig, G.; Hoffman, R.; Oliven, A.; Rowe, J.M.; Brenner, B. Hemostatic Balance on the Surface of Leukemic Cells: The Role of Tissue Factor and Urokinase Plasminogen Activator Receptor. *Haematologica* **2005**, *90*, 1549–1556.
19. Dubois, C.; Schlageter, M.H.; de Gentile, A.; Guidez, F.; Balitrand, N.; Toubert, M.E.; Krawice, I.; Fenaux, P.; Castaigne, S.; Najean, Y. Hematopoietic Growth Factor Expression and Atra Sensitivity in Acute Promyelocytic Blast Cells. *Blood* **1994**, *83*, 3264–3270.
20. Holig, K.; Moog, R. Leukocyte Depletion by Therapeutic Leukocytapheresis in Patients with Leukemia. *Transfus. Med. Hemother.* **2012**, *39*, 241–245. [CrossRef]
21. Novotny, J.R.; Muller-Beissenhirtz, H.; Herget-Rosenthal, S.; Kribben, A.; Duhrsen, U. Grading of Symptoms in Hyperleukocytic Leukaemia: A Clinical Model for the Role of Different Blast Types and Promyelocytes in the Development of Leukostasis Syndrome. *Eur. J. Haematol.* **2005**, *74*, 501–510. [CrossRef]

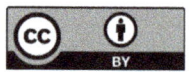 © 2019 by the authors. Licensee MDPI, Basel, Switzerland. This article is an open access article distributed under the terms and conditions of the Creative Commons Attribution (CC BY) license (http://creativecommons.org/licenses/by/4.0/).

MDPI
St. Alban-Anlage 66
4052 Basel
Switzerland
Tel. +41 61 683 77 34
Fax +41 61 302 89 18
www.mdpi.com

Brain Sciences Editorial Office
E-mail: brainsci@mdpi.com
www.mdpi.com/journal/brainsci